still

still

A MEMOIR OF LOVE, LOSS, AND MOTHERHOOD

EMMA HANSEN

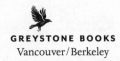

GREYSTONE BOOKS
Vancouver / Berkeley

20 21 22 23 24   5 4 3 2 1

Greystone Books Ltd.
greystonebooks.com

Cataloguing data available from Library and Archives Canada
ISBN 978-1-77164-391-7 (pbk.)
ISBN 978-1-77164-392-4 (epub)

Editing by Paula Ayer
Copyediting by Antonia Banyard
Proofreading by Jennifer Stewart
Cover and text design by Belle Wuthrich
Cover artwork by Alana Hansen

Printed and bound in Canada on ancient-forest-friendly paper by Friesens

"The Waking," copyright © 1966 and renewed 1994 by Beatrice Lushington; from *Collected Poems* by Theodore Roethke. Used by permission of Doubleday, an imprint of the Knopf Doubleday Publishing Group, a division of Penguin Random House LLC. All rights reserved.

Greystone Books gratefully acknowledges the Musqueam, Squamish, and Tsleil-Waututh peoples on whose land our office is located.

Greystone Books thanks the Canada Council for the Arts, the British Columbia Arts Council, the Province of British Columbia through the Book Publishing Tax Credit, and the Government of Canada for supporting our publishing activities.

Canadä

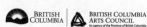

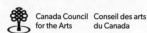

For Aaron and Everett
In honor, celebration,
and memory of Reid

THIS IS MY story, as I remember it, allowing that time and grief have rendered some memories unreachable. Some events have been compressed or reordered; conversations have been reconstructed from memory. Passages from my blog and social media have been incorporated to stay true to the grief of those seasons. Some names have been changed to protect the anonymity of those persons, and some have been kept as they are in real life. I acknowledge that if your gender, ethnicity, sexuality, religion, experiences, or beliefs are different than mine, what is written on these pages might not always resonate. If this is true, I say: I see you, your story is important in its differences and similarities, and I hope you feel supported by this book as a whole. In all ways, I have attempted to honor the roles that the members of my far-reaching community have had in my journey. I write with gratitude for these connections. Though this is my story, I am not alone in it.

I wake to sleep, and take my waking slow.
I feel my fate in what I cannot fear.
I learn by going where I have to go.

—THEODORE ROETHKE, "The Waking"

Prologue

SEE HIM AGAIN in November. It's the first time. The little gray-and-white chevron cardigan we'd bought for him is still rolled up at the wrists. His hat sits a little too far back on his head, letting wisps of black hair escape from underneath. His cheeks are flushed red through his porcelain skin.

I walk toward him, through the crisp winter air, through the backyard of my childhood home. I circle the edge of the pool and notice the muddle of leaves and worms sitting in its depths. The grand Douglas fir stands tall at the back of the yard, but the shrubs growing wildly around it are naked in their state of rest. Under the canopy of the fir, in the spot next to the large, wayward root where our late dog Magnus used to lie, Reid sits in his car seat, eyes closed. Even though time has passed, he is still a newborn, as he was that single day in April when we gazed upon his face. All evidence of his passing has been erased. I'm dreaming, of course I'm dreaming, but it feels more real than anything I've experienced before.

I am visiting him, as one visits a grave, and I have brought him a flower, white and blooming in my grasp, its petals dropping as I walk closer to him. It looks like an oleander, beautiful and poisonous, but that can't be right. My sister Alana is with me and she takes photos as I place it softly on his chest.

We leave him and walk inside the long-abandoned home. A waning sun shines through the hall windows, and dust glitters in its beams. We wave our hands in front of us, sending the dust on a dance through the air, and clear a path to the smallest room in the house, the one that was mine for most of our years here. My sister and I sit next to each other on the bed and look through the photos we've taken. Then something captures my attention. When I zoom in for a closer look, I see that Reid's eyes are open, and he's looking directly at the camera.

I nearly drop the phone. We jump up and run back to the tree to where he's still sitting, his eyes now wide and focused. My breath catches in my throat. They are a beautiful shade of pale blue.

We swoon over him, taking photos and capturing videos. My dad comes out from the house in his wheelchair and places Reid on his lap, spins him around the pool, looks into his eyes. Then Aaron is there, holding him in the crook of his arm. Just like at his birth, only this time Reid is looking at him too, kicking and stretching his long arms up toward his father's face. We invite the rest of our family and friends—the ones who held him seven months earlier—and the scene around the pool morphs into a party, everyone talking and laughing and passing Reid back and forth, celebrating that he is here.

Eventually the guests fade away. When the sun finally sets and just the two of us are left, sitting side by side, I sense that it's nearly time for him to go. I don't want to move, fearing that the tiniest shift will erase him from my presence. So we sit under the glow of the full moon rising above and our breath paints the air before us. I marvel at how such a simple moment can bring me such joy. I am only sitting in the cold of the night with my son at my side, but *he is breathing.*

"Where have you been?" I ask.

"I've been right here." The words come from him, but he doesn't so much speak them to me as *into* me, and his hand moves to rest over his heart. "I've been near you this whole time."

"Do you know how much I love you?" I brush his hair up off his forehead.

A smile spreads across his face, revealing a single dimple on his left cheek, like mine.

● ☾ ●

I NEVER KNOW when I'll sense Reid's presence. It isn't in a toothbrush left behind or a frequently worn item of clothing. It's in the absences that I feel him most. It's everywhere that I had imagined he'd one day be.

For me, he is more than his body. I knew the soul, not the flesh. When I look at photos of him, I miss him, but not in the same way I miss him when I look at photos of myself pregnant.

He is a feeling. He is a feeling more than anything because of the simple fact that he died before he was born. Because he was stillborn. He is not defined by this, but the definition matters. I was meant to be his portal, the one that would lead him from his world into ours, but he left for another world, one altogether foreign to me. His life was supposed to start with his birth, but I have learned that his story began long before then, just as I have learned that it will continue long after. They were gifts, his life and his death. I never really lived before either.

I

I T IS A TUESDAY, the last one of my pregnancy. March is rounding the corner into April, and the transition from winter to spring has begun. My mother and I are out for lunch on West Fourth Avenue after a walk by the ocean, with the city on the other side of the bay, lambent in the soft northern sun and decorated by the earliest signs of cherry blossoms. In the restaurant, we sit in a narrow booth—my belly pressed up against the table edge, not quite able to fit in the space provided—and wait for our food to arrive. I shift uncomfortably in my seat but don't have the energy to bother suggesting we move.

My mother has two speeds: racehorse fast or complete standstill. There is no in-between. Most of my childhood memories of her are of her back, with me toddling behind, trying to match her pace. My father, by contrast, has only one setting: always moving, yet somehow always late. I inherited that trait from him.

It's nice to catch my mom at a slower pace than usual, and I relish the new ease our relationship has gained during my pregnancy. We were never especially close when I was growing up. Desperate for my independence, I spent most of my adolescent years trying to push her away, until I moved to New York after high school. Living under the same roof was never good for either of us. Living abroad had helped, but this baby is helping the most.

"Are you nervous?" she asks, putting her phone facedown on the table.

"What, about the birth?" I think about it for a moment. "Actually, no," I answer honestly. I'm really not all that nervous. During our birthing classes, we've gone over things as thoroughly as I figure is possible and I know what to expect. "We don't have much of a birth plan," I continue. "I'm pretty open to whatever is needed."

She nods, "That's a good way to go into it." Then, tucking a wayward strand of red hair behind her ear, she muses, "I wonder if he'll come this weekend? Near his due date?"

"Wouldn't that be something?" Imagining it then, I smile. My due date is this Saturday, and early deliveries run in the family. I'm already further along in my pregnancy than my mother or grandmother had ever been in theirs.

The waiter arrives with our salads, and we continue to talk and laugh and wonder about all that is to come.

After our meal, my mom and I plan to meet up again on Friday for another walk along the ocean. She'll call me after her hair appointment. I'll call her sooner if there are any signs of impending labor. I return home to take a nap and fold the laundry in the nursery. Little clothes in neutral colors lie spread across the floor: a onesie that wraps around and ties at the side; mittens made to look like the paws of a bear; a sun hat that seems enormous in comparison, meant for the summer months when he'll be older. I imagine the stains of milk and mud and berries these bits of fabric will collect, and all the things we'll do together fill my mind—these tiny clothes from the growing pile before me seeming to come to life in my daydreams of what's ahead.

Aaron comes home later in the afternoon to find me at the computer. I'm writing a post titled "Pregnancy-Approved Smoothies" on the blog I started last year, as a way to fill the gaps between my modeling jobs when we were still living in New York. He kisses me hello as I hit *publish*.

"How about mushroom risotto for dinner?" he asks, heading to the kitchen.

"I was going to make a salad," I reply. If it were up to me, we'd eat salad every night. It's why Aaron often does the cooking.

"Sure, salad is an important *part* of a meal," he teases, and I throw a pillow at him. He laughs sweetly, then peers into the nursery I've finished organizing, taking in the car seat, the stroller, the storage unit full of children's books and folded swaddles and toys.

"Wow." He beams. "We're really ready for him!"

I'll never tire of his passion. The way he is all in when something excites him. Like the time he came home to our New York apartment saying, "You'll never guess what I found!" then proudly revealed the pile of wood he had rescued from a construction site dump, which he proceeded to transform into beautiful hand-built seating for our patio. Or when he announced, "I've learned another language!" and pointed at the cryptic type on his computer screen, patiently explaining how he had taught himself the software coding that would become his career. Aaron is a living, breathing database full of information. If there is anything I ever wonder, I don't need to look it up—he will know. It was one of the things that first made me fall in love with him.

I go to the doorway and wrap my arms around him as we gaze into the nursery together. I think back to nine months ago, and my anxious tears when those two pink lines first appeared on the pregnancy test. We hadn't been trying to avoid pregnancy, but at twenty-four and twenty-six, it wasn't exactly part of our plan to have kids this young. But Aaron was all in for this too.

"We can do this," he reassured me after I'd given him the big news. "I'm excited."

And I believed him. And I'm excited too.

That evening, Aaron and I head out to our appointment with the local community birth program. We chose the program, run by a team of doctors, midwives, and doulas, at the end of my first trimester. Being young and healthy, I didn't feel the need to be under the care of an obstetrician, but being cautious, I wasn't comfortable with the idea of a home birth either. This program seemed like the perfect medium. We like their philosophy of restoring pregnancy and birth to the community-oriented experiences they had been traditionally.

The way the program works, our prenatal appointments are piggybacked onto a two-hour group lesson with other couples who are due around the same time as us. We are the youngest couple there by nearly a decade. The first day we walked in, we both felt shy about our youth. But we quickly realized that everyone else was just as lost as we were, and over the months we've bonded with the other families. Most of us are expecting our first child, and the weekly progress of our pregnancies is an intimate experience we've shared. Some of the other women and I go to prenatal yoga together on the weekends, and I've taken a particular liking to the French-Canadian couple who often sit next to us.

The familiar faces are all there tonight, along with three new attendees. A few of the couples have given birth already and are there with their newborns. They are so small, their scrunched-up faces looking even smaller beneath the layers their parents have swaddled them with. "We don't know how much to dress them in!" they exclaim. I can't imagine how completely their lives have changed, but I watch in wonder as they navigate the needy cries of these tiny humans. Aaron and I gape at each other, communicating without words. All of a sudden, everything seems to be happening very quickly.

As we're called away from the group for our checkup with our midwife, I think again about how lucky I've been to have a healthy pregnancy, free of complications. This is in contrast to the complicated birth stories my mother has to tell. With me, the oldest, my mother developed a liver disorder called ICP and had to be induced at thirty-eight weeks. With my middle sister, Alana, my mother slipped on ice at thirty weeks and ruptured her membranes, then developed gestational diabetes while on bed rest, delivering by cesarean a few weeks later when the baby went into distress. Alana, born at a relatively healthy five pounds, only spent a few days in the neonatal intensive care unit under the bili lights for jaundice. With my youngest sister, Rebecca, my mother had dangerously high blood pressure and required another emergency cesarean at thirty-three weeks. Born at only three pounds, Rebecca spent time in the NICU too.

So I was expecting complicated. Because of my mother's history, I've been monitored a little more closely than normal—borderline tests redone and a few extra ordered when necessary. But at each appointment my unremarkable results have been attributed to my youth and active lifestyle. The baby is always lively, his heartbeat is strong, his growth on track. With every passing week I've grown more convinced of the assurances of the birth team that everything will continue to be normal.

We step into the sectioned-off area near the front where our midwife, Fiona, is waiting. She asks us how we're doing. I say we're fine, just fine, and ask if she can guess the baby's weight. The only thing I am a little bit nervous about is him fitting out of me. My hips are narrow, and I am not entirely convinced a baby can exit through them. Surely a lot of bones will have to shift. Fiona laughs and places her hands on my belly, feeling around our baby's body and smiling at the nudges he gives her. She estimates seven and a half pounds, and I let out a sigh of relief. I can do seven pounds.

"Of course," she says, "it's only my best guess." Sensing that I need reassurance, she adds, "I will say, I'm usually very close." She grabs the Doppler off the top of her desk to monitor his heart rate. "Let's have a listen, shall we?"

I know the drill. I lift up my shirt and watch the wand slide the jelly down the slope of my bump. Immediately, we hear the *whoosh, whoosh, whoosh.*

"All is good! What a chill baby," Fiona notes, moving the Doppler around a bit.

I listen to the sound of his heartbeat. Like a galloping horse. The rhythmic melody circles around the room. But a tiny voice speaks up from the back of my mind through the noise. *Is it a bit slower than usual?* I shush it. Everything is fine. We are fine. Nothing bad can happen at this point. We are nearly there, almost home. The voice goes away and I return to listening to the beating of his heart. A little longer, I suggest. *Whoosh, whoosh, whoosh.*

2

SLOWLY, HEAVILY, I blink open my eyes. Looking to the still-made sheets where Aaron's body should be, I rub a hand over my swollen belly, waiting for a kick. Aaron must have slept on the couch again. He's been doing that on the nights when sleep doesn't come. He gets too hot. And, apparently, pregnancy makes me snore.

I look to the clock. It's 9:31 AM, Friday, April 3, the day before our due date, which falls on a total lunar eclipse, a full blood moon. Today is also Good Friday, and for weeks now I've been greeted by Easter decorations whenever I leave home. I've spent my pregnancy preparing for an Easter baby, so they've made our child's anticipated birth even more real.

Last night, Aaron and I walked to the drugstore on the corner to buy some Cadbury Eggs to satisfy an urgent craving. When we reached the till to pay we were greeted by a friendly woman with happy cheeks and wiry black hair. "Oh my god! When are you due?" she shouted upon seeing my belly. I smiled at her and rubbed the little feet poking at my side as I replied that my due date was on Saturday. She clucked and said she would be flat on her back at home if she were two days away from having her baby. I don't know why, but hearing that made me proud. Even if I was only out to buy myself a family-sized bag of chocolate, I felt powerful in that moment.

Fully awake now, I roll over to my left side and gently press myself up to sit. The bed creaks in protest, and so do my aching joints. I pivot my body to face the edge and extend a leg to reach for the stepping stool. With an arched back, I cling to the sheets to get a few inches further and wrap my toes around the wooden rail to drag it closer. Aaron built the bed from scratch last year and I demanded it be enormous, the biggest bed he could make. It seems a little excessive now, given that I need a small ladder to get my large belly in and out of it.

I grab my robe and tie it loosely around my body; I have been mostly sleeping in underwear, since even Aaron's shirts don't fit me anymore. My toe joints crack against the hardwood as I make my way to the kitchen in search of breakfast. Once there, I peek my head around the wall of the passthrough and see Aaron at the desk. He has the day off from work for the holiday weekend and is busy doing taxes. I fight the urge to remind him he needs to have them finished by tomorrow, our due date, like he promised.

"Morning," I manage through a yawn.

He turns around and flashes a smile. "Oh, hi!" Then, directed toward my belly: "Good morning!"

I bend over to kiss his forehead and he returns one to our baby, then I shuffle back to the kitchen for food. I settle on granola, my staple over the last trimester. I bring the bowl to the bedroom and climb back into bed. Balancing the bowl on my belly, I crunch on oat clusters and browse through the various apps on my phone.

Then I hear the voice again, that of a worried mother. It has spoken only a few times during my pregnancy: when I noticed a speckle of blood at five weeks; at our anatomy ultrasound when it showed something unexpected; when my midwife suggested further testing to rule out gestational hypertension; and earlier this week at our appointment when the heartbeat seemed a little slower than usual. Now I hear it again, bellowing at me: *He hasn't kicked yet!*

I shush it. Everything is fine; everything is always fine. I feel ridiculous for even entertaining the worry. I climb out of bed to grab my computer. I think about opening up Netflix to watch *Parenthood*, the show I started earlier this week, in an effort to distract myself. Lauren Graham is in it and as a *Gilmore Girls* fan that's about all it needed to win my love. But the voice only grows louder. *Why hasn't he moved?*

I grab my phone. It's 10:05 AM. I quickly search "Brittany" and type:

So close to our due dates! How are you feeling?

I put the phone on the pillow and wait. Brittany, my blond-haired, bright-eyed, full-of-life friend, is due the day after me, April 5, and we've talked nearly every day of our pregnancies.

10:42 AM. My phone buzzes. Brittany's reply reads:

I can't believe it!!!!!!! I am feeling still pregnant. How are you?

How am I? *I'm freaking out. I can't shake this feeling that something is wrong,* I type, then hit delete until the text field is clear. It doesn't help; the feeling persists. I type again:

I feel ya! I'm trying to not be too impatient and enjoy these last days but man I just want to meet this little guy!!! I hit send.

My stomach churns, then prickles nervously the way it does in moments of heightened anxiety. It won't be settled with pastimes or entertainment; I need to do something. I reach for my home Doppler—which I purchased in my first trimester—from my bedside table drawer and turn it on. I hit the power button, squeeze the jelly onto the wand, and press it to my belly. I wait for the familiar *whoosh, whoosh, whoosh* but there is nothing, just static. I move it around. Still nothing. I pull out the instructions and try to read them, but the words blur together on the page.

"Aaron!" I yell.

I hear the screech of his chair pushing back. He appears in the doorway and after one look at me says, "What's wrong?"

"I can't remember how to use this." I hold the Doppler up by the wand. "I haven't felt him move yet this morning and now I can't find his heartbeat."

He sits down on the edge of the bed and calmly reads the instructions—he is inherently logical, he will figure it out. After flipping a switch he squirts more jelly on the wand and gently holds it below my belly button. Static. He fiddles with some dials and slides the wand down lower. More static. He takes my hand and holds it for a moment. Then he gives it a little squeeze and asks, hopefully, "Maybe it's broken?"

I know it isn't.

I throw myself off the bed and run to get the magnet off our fridge with the emergency numbers for our medical team. I plant myself down on the exercise ball in the center of the living room floor and ask Aaron to get me a glass of orange juice, a boost of sugar for the baby. As I dial the numbers to page the doctor on call, I bounce in gentle circles and repeat aloud: "Wake up baby, wake up baby, wake up baby." Clockwise and then counterclockwise. Back and forth.

The phone rings for what seems like much longer than normal before I am greeted by the medical receptionist, who puts me through to the midwife on call. "I haven't felt my baby move yet this morning," I repeat. The gentle voice of the midwife speaks calmly into my ear.

"Hi Emma, this is Tess," she begins. "Have you tried drinking some cold orange juice? Lying down for an hour?"

"Yes," I lie. Not about the orange juice, but about the lying down; I'm not willing to wait an hour. I bounce up and down. "He usually moves as soon as I wake up. This has never happened before."

Tess calmly tells us to come in to get monitored, assuring us that babies tend to slow down right before delivery. I hold on to those words as tightly as I can as I gather my things.

"Should we bring our hospital bags?" I ask Aaron, struggling with a toppling Ugg boot.

"No," he answers, grabbing my shoe to steady it for me to step into. "If we need them, I can come back and get them. It's not like the baby is coming right now, right?"

Aaron and I run out of the door and drive to the hospital, ten minutes away. We arrive at eleven thirty. As we walk through the Labor and Delivery doors for the first time, I keep thinking that this isn't how it should be. I'm probably just over-worrying; there is nothing wrong with our boy. But by the time we reach Admitting my panic is rising—I still haven't felt him move.

"What brings you in today?" A nurse greets us with a smile.

"I haven't felt our baby move yet this morning," I repeat for what feels like the hundredth time that day, but with more urgency. "I called ahead and spoke with the midwife on call, Tess."

As the nurse shuffles through some papers my eyes lock with those of a woman down the hall. Her blond hair is pulled back tightly and the tops of her cheekbones catch the light just so. In one hand she holds a Starbucks cup and with the other she is rubbing the back of her laboring client, in a hospital gown beside her. A doula. I know it instantly.

"Are you with the birth program?" the woman asks.

I nod.

"Who's your doula?" A slightly annoyed look crosses her face. "And where is she?"

"Jill," I answer. "But I'm not in labor. So—"

The conversation stops there because the nurse is now directing us toward the registration desk. I look back at the doula and smile, as if to say, "thank you for caring." Later, I'll remember this. The last smile *before*.

The administrative worker asks me to sit, takes our information, and attaches a hospital band to my wrist. Another nurse brings us to the side and pulls out a Doppler. I read the name on her tag: Hilary. As she works on the machine I look up to study her. She is sweet, with strawberry-blond hair that frames her slender face in tight little waves. She keeps her lips pursed in a straight line.

She reaches for the jelly. As she shakes it onto the probe, she asks, "What position is baby usually in?"

"Head down, back along the left, feet up in my right ribs." I rub the curve of his back down my side. "But maybe he's moved?"

"Okay, let's take a look," she says. "Lift up your shirt."

I fold the bottom of my black-and-gray-striped tee to the top of my belly and sit back in the chair. Hilary places the probe below my belly button, to the left, then glides it over my skin slowly, looking for the heartbeat. It must be only a minute, but it's the longest minute of my life. I watch Hilary's face the entire time, all the while clutching Aaron's hand, and in those sixty seconds her expression goes from fresh and confident to very panicked. I know then that something is terribly wrong.

She switches off the machine. "You know what? These things break all the time. Let's just get you into a room and hook you up to the better monitors." We follow quickly behind her. In the room, she instructs me to get on the bed. Her hands tremble and she bites her lip as she fidgets to get the straps around my belly and hook up my own pulse monitor. Immediately, the monitor shows 130 bpm, which would be a relief were it not in sync with my own heart rate. This sets off the monitor's alarms. Hilary tries to silence them, but they ring all around us. The rhythmic beating of my heart quickens, echoing out of the speakers. The monitors show 150 bpm. The alarms continue to sound.

Tess, the midwife I spoke to on the phone, appears. I am struggling to breathe.

"There, there," she hushes. "What's wrong?" She manages to turn off the alarms and takes my hand, trying to get me to calm down, but I can't.

"They can't find his heartbeat!" I gasp, and then start to sob.

"That sounds like one, doesn't it? One fifty?" She turns to Hilary, who shakes her head.

"No, that's hers," she says.

Aaron meets my gaze and we hold it as a flurry of activity erupts around us. For that moment time stands still, just for a second, and we brace ourselves for what is to come.

"We're going to do an ultrasound," someone declares. "Just to check."

A resident wheels in the portable ultrasound machine. She repeats what Hilary said earlier, that it will be much quicker at picking up his heartbeat. She turns on the screen, finds his heart, and pauses. I see that it is still.

I will his heart to start beating again. *Just beat, one more time.* The resident asks for the attending doctor, Dr. L., as she keeps the probe pressed firmly into my side. Dr. L. arrives, and the resident asks for confirmation that she has the ultrasound positioned on the heart.

"Yes," he replies. And then, "Turn on the blood flow imaging."

The screen doesn't change. Dr. L. nods solemnly at the resident. And then she speaks the worst words I'll ever hear:

"Okay. I have the ultrasound focused on his heart now. Do you see that?" She points to a spot in the middle of the screen. "It's not moving. And there's no red and blue to signify blood flow. I'm so sorry, but your baby is dead."

Suddenly, it's as if I'm removed from everything, a bystander on the outskirts of someone else's trauma. I see us collapse into each other's arms, breathless and sobbing. I see Aaron drape himself over my belly, hear him beg for a kick. I see the nurses and doctors that have been buzzing around us slowly trickle out of the room. All I can feel is my heart, how it threatens to escape my chest, and my throat, which houses foreign cries. Everything else seems to have fallen away.

I look at the clock and realize that it is almost one. I am supposed to be meeting my mom for our walk. Then the thought hits me that we'll have to tell our families. I tell Aaron, and he takes my phone. I gather my hands in front of my face and whimper into the curves of them as he dials my mother's number.

"Amanda? It's Aaron." He pauses. I can't hear her, but I sense her confusion anyway.

"We're at the hospital. I think you should come. They can't find Reid's heartbeat." He uses our favorite of the names we chose for our baby. Then I hear the muffled panic of my mother's raised voice.

"No. No," he chokes. "They can't find it. He's gone."

He makes more calls, each one breaking my heart into a million more pieces, each one constructing a new level of shock. I don't think I can face the pain on our families' faces, though I know I will need their support more than anything.

My mother bursts into the room with an air of authority and asks the nurse what is happening. She fixes things, my mother, and she is ready to fix this too. But she can't, not now. I just wail in her arms and tell her that it's too late, that our baby is dead.

And then, for a moment, I can't cry. I sit there and I stare. I stare at my quiet belly and repeat the words to myself slowly, trying to understand. *Our baby is dead.* Beneath my skin is the body of our child, and somehow that body has to come out. I am sure that they will put me under and cut him from me.

In the throes of trauma, time moves strangely. It can't have been more than five minutes, surely, but somehow my father, sisters, and in-laws have joined us. But my in-laws would have had to drive in from the Fraser Valley, over an hour away. It makes no sense, but little does right now.

With our loved ones by our side we let the doctors back in to talk us through what we need to do next. Dr. L. appears in the doorway and says he will take us to get a detailed ultrasound to try to determine the cause of death.

"Do you want a wheelchair?" he asks.

I refuse. I'll walk, of course I'll walk. But as soon as I take a step I realize it is a terrible mistake. My body feels different and even though nothing has changed physically from this morning—I walked to the car, I walked into the hospital—I am hyperaware of the lifeless body inside me, shifting from side to side as I move. Perhaps that was why they offered. I make my legs move anyway.

We walk through the hospital to the ultrasound wing, the same one we went through twenty weeks ago to find out we were having a boy. We walk past couples standing in the hallway, then couples sitting in chairs waiting for their turn. They quickly look away from our grief-stricken faces, but their knuckles turn white as they hold each other's hands a little tighter. We are their worst nightmare. They don't know exactly what has happened to us, but they can guess. And they know, without a doubt, that they do not want to end up here.

We enter the ultrasound room. It is dark and no one turns on the lights. I fumble my way to the bed and Aaron helps me onto the fragile paper sprawled across it. Then Dr. L. is talking. He asks us if he should turn on the patients' screen. "Do you want to watch?"

I turn to Aaron for an answer. How can we decide? I am sure I will regret it if I don't. But how can I watch that screen? A black-and-white movie, frozen on the edge of possibility, forever without color. In the end, I look.

After some searching, Dr. L. sees that my placenta is pale and that there is a tiny bit of fluid around the baby's heart. But both of those things are also common postmortem, he says, so they don't necessarily indicate the cause of death. He says that we most likely will never find out what happened, that it's a sad part of life that sometimes babies just pass for no medical reason, and being dragged through months of tests and autopsies will be more painful than we realize right now. But, he says, the choice is absolutely ours. I am inclined to take his advice, even understanding that without an autopsy, we'll probably never know what happened.

He leaves us by saying that the chance of anything like this happening to us again would be like getting hit by lightning twice. We shouldn't fear the future.

Back in the assessment room, a new obstetrician comes in to review our options. All of them involve me having to deliver our dead baby vaginally, something I am completely unprepared to hear. The idea of laboring, which I was so calm about before, terrifies me now. I'm not ready. I want it to be finished, but I also don't want it to start. How strange that something I anticipated with such joyful ease, I now view with such fright.

Why haven't they offered me a C-section yet, offered to medicate me into a deep sleep? I just want to close my eyes and wake up with it all over. A part of me hopes that during the process, there's a chance I won't wake up at all. But I don't ask. Maybe because I can't fathom how any woman can get through birthing her lifeless child, either vaginally or surgically.

I am given the option of either an oxytocin drip to induce labor right away, or a Cervidil insert to soften my cervix. I choose the latter so that we can go home to rest and prepare for what comes next.

The obstetrician unwraps the Cervidil and reaches a hand inside of me. I struggle away from her to the top of the bed, in pain. She holds my hips in place with her free hand to stop me from squirming and reaches in further still. She simply tells me, "You need to get it right up there against the cervix." Then she pulls out her hand, takes the glove off, and continues, "It'll likely take a few doses of this, so come by in the morning to get your next one. They might start you on the oxytocin if you've progressed."

A nurse with white hair and soft eyes comes in and hands me a pair of hospital underwear and a pad, in case of bleeding if my cervix starts to dilate. She has a gentleness about her, one that suggests she might have done this before, cared for others through losses.

"But our due date is tomorrow," I tell her as a silent plea for her to change what is happening. Can't she undo his death if I make it clear how impossible it is? He lived for thirty-nine weeks and six days in my womb. How is it that he stopped living just one day before his due date? *One day.*

"I know, dear," she says as she helps me off the bed. "I'm so sorry."

I put the mesh underwear on in the bathroom, avoiding the mirror as I do.

● ☾ ●

IT WAS DECIDED that we weren't in any state to drive home. My mother-in-law, Annette, waited behind to take us in our car while the others went ahead to our apartment. I don't remember leaving the hospital, but we end up in our car. Annette takes the speed bumps slowly and it makes me wonder if she senses the pain they'll cause me, each bump startling the body at rest inside of mine.

It's five thirty when we walk into the apartment. Hank, Aaron's dad, is standing off to the side near the corner window in our living room. My parents are in the hallway, and my two younger sisters, Alana and Rebecca, are sitting on the couch—they are both university students, and I think of how they should be studying for their finals right now. Hanah, Aaron's sister and one of my best friends, and her boyfriend, Carson, are on their way. Aaron's brothers are out of town—Derek on a missions trip in India, Levi at school in Ontario—and we're told they're booking flights to come back as soon as possible.

Arriving home feels like tumbling into a twilight zone— like we're stuck in a past that no longer fits, with the future lingering just out of reach. Everything is exactly as we left it just a few hours earlier, except the dishes have been washed and our living room tidied.

My mother tells me later that they stressed about what to do to prepare for our arrival. Should they put away the baby items? Do our laundry? Hide evidence of my pregnancy? In the end, they knew that they couldn't just wipe all signs of our child from existence. So they left everything as it was—including the nursery door, slightly ajar. Once they were exhausted from conversation and tears they looked for something to watch on our TV. Unable to figure out how to summon Netflix into view, they rifled through our towering stack of DVDs in search of something happy to distract them. They ended up pulling out the disc Aaron had made of our trip to Disneyland, a year after we'd started dating. Tears poured out of them as they watched us on the screen: happy, naive, carefree teenagers. We rode rollercoasters and laughed as the cart turned this way and that, kissing for the camera on the upward climbs. Would we ever be the same? they wondered out loud, to no one in particular.

In the haze that surrounds the hours after that resident wheeled in the ultrasound, there are pockets of dreamlike clarity. I feel vividly aware of my senses as I sit down on the couch and fold my legs up beneath me. I am mindful not to move, not wanting to feel his lifeless body stir inside of me. The sensation makes me ill, and then incredibly guilty in turn. My belly is still round, but it has changed. I'm not sure what to do, but I can't let it be real yet. I don't know where to put my hands. It feels wrong to place them on my stomach, so they fall awkwardly at my sides. Someone hands me a bowl of tomato soup and tells me to eat. As I sit there, slowly and methodically lifting the spoon to my mouth, I hear my mother and Annette in the kitchen around the corner, whispering.

"I think she's in shock," Annette says to my mom.

I mull that over. Am I not acting how I'm supposed to? How should you behave while waiting to birth a child who is already dead? While waiting to gaze upon the face of that child for the very first time, knowing that they will soon fade from memory? There is no making sense of the unfathomable, and so I sit. I sit and I eat tomato soup and I watch *Friends* on the television. I'll never be able to do any of those things in the same way after.

I don't actually watch. Instead, I am stuck in my own mind, traveling back to my childhood. I'm in sixth grade at a new school with new teachers, and already they've pegged me for the perfectionist I am. We're at an end-of-school weekend retreat for my year, some hundred of us, and on the last day they give out satirical awards to some of the students. I win the "Failure to Fail" award. They have me come up in front of all my peers to attempt something that simply isn't doable: shove a box full of crackers in my mouth and then whistle. I am determined to prove them wrong, and as I blow with all my might, a cloud of crumbs bursts out before me. The room erupts in laughter, and I feel my face flush red with embarrassment. I have only failed to do what is obviously impossible, but all I see is that I have failed. It is the first time I can recall feeling so devastated.

I have failed many times since then. Stumbled and crumpled and collapsed in defeat. But as I sit here now I see all of my past failures as trivial compared to this, because this time I failed and a life was lost. *Our baby is dead.* I keep repeating that over and over and over again in my mind until the words mean nothing to me. How will Aaron ever forgive me? How will I ever forgive myself?

It is an inexplicable feeling to carry death inside you when the very concept of pregnancy is so explicitly connected to life. To be in a room surrounded by family mourning a soul that has departed when the body has not. He is still here. He is with us. And he has to come out. You can't bury a body in utero, can't cremate remains that exist in the in-between. Instead, you have to do the impossible. Somehow, it must be done.

3

LESS THAN AN hour after we get home my first contractions start. Hanah has just arrived with Carson, and her confusion over my still-full belly is palpable. Annette called her when Hanah was on a ferry to Vancouver Island. As she heard the news, she slid down the cabin wall and came apart on the floor, gasping for air. Somehow, she is here. She has never been one to hide emotion, and I can see how hard she is trying now. I feel the toll this is taking on her, and for a moment it distracts me from my own pain.

The rushes roll in gently at first—every three minutes, but manageable with a little focused breathing. My body is ready. My mom sits next to me on the couch, careful not to touch me, but her presence is grounding. *Friends* plays on in the background.

I pick up my phone and open up the contraction timer app I downloaded months ago in preparation. Every time I hit *record* my mom looks to me and asks, "Another one? So soon?"

By nine PM I can no longer divert my focus with TV and deep breaths. It's starting. I ask everyone to leave, though the goodbyes are a blur.

Aaron is running a bath behind me, and I am bent over the counter riding out another contraction. We paged the hospital a few minutes ago, asking if I should be in so much pain so soon. Susie, the new midwife on call with our birth program, told us the Cervidil could sometimes cause intense and false contractions. "Take it out," she suggested. "Just like you would a tampon. Then hop in the bath. The warm water should help you relax." Before hanging up, she added, "Come back in the morning for another dose, but only once you've slept. Really do try to get some rest."

I climb into the tub to soak as Aaron props himself up on the ledge. We try to talk through what is happening.

"Maybe we'll be one of those inexplicable medical marvels and he will come out screaming," Aaron says.

Yes, maybe that's it. I've read the articles that sometimes circulate on Facebook about babies they thought were dead who were placed on their mothers' chests, then suddenly cried out. I am skeptical, but I don't want to be. We believe in God—a God that is good. We believe that miracles are possible through Him. What is that belief for, if it can't help us now?

So we start to pray. We pray that He will save our child, bring him back to life, change what has happened. We believe that He can. And just in case, wanting to cover all of our bases, we pray that the doctors are wrong and that he isn't dead. Surely, he will be born and he'll take his first breath and everything will make sense again. I want to hold out hope that our miracle is within reach, that the fact that our baby has died on the same day Jesus was crucified is significant. *There's something to that, isn't there?*

Only that bellowing voice of the fiercely protective mother is gone; she speaks solely in moans now. Making it through this experience with our baby alive doesn't really seem like an option. But how desperately I want to believe that it is.

The bath isn't helping. I turn the water back on, all the way to hot, hoping it will burn away the pain. Having spent the better part of a year soaking in lukewarm baths to keep our baby safe, I am shocked by the heat.

"When I was pregnant—" I start, wanting to explain to Aaron what I am feeling. But I stop, not sure how to continue. Am I still pregnant? I remember the saying, "You can't be just a little bit pregnant." We think of pregnancy as a very clear "you are or you aren't" situation, so much so that it's inspired the idiom meaning there's no gray area or uncertainty. But what about when you are still carrying a child, but not a living one? I shudder at the thought and don't continue my sentence. Aaron doesn't press me for more.

Soon, I can't make it through my contractions without clutching Aaron's hand, fighting back against the force of them. We had decided that we would try to labor at our place for as long as possible—that was one of our only hopes from the start of this pregnancy and we wanted to stick to our basic birth plan as much as possible. But we need help. Aaron calls our doula, Jill—he has been texting her with updates since we were in the hospital—and asks her to come over. My contractions are now just over a minute and a half apart, lasting for sixty seconds. That leaves me thirty seconds of rest in between them, and it isn't enough. Nothing could ever be enough for this. "I can't do this without pain relief anymore," I moan. "We need to go in."

Aaron looks relieved to have something to do. He calls Jill again and tells her to meet us at the hospital instead, then gathers our things by the door. By 10:50 PM we are off.

Ten minutes later, we are back at Admitting. A nurse greets us, smiling. "Are you having contractions?" she asks cheerfully.

"I am," I start, pausing to breathe through one. She waits, and I squeeze my eyes shut as I sway. "But we're here under different circumstances," I continue. "If you look up my name, you'll see."

She looks at me from behind the desk, clearly confused, and asks again if I am in labor. "You'll just need to sit in the waiting room and we'll call when we have time to admit you."

I can't believe her. How does she not know what happened? How has the whole world not stopped to grieve with us? I shout at her that my baby died, that I was induced, that I need to be seen right away. I am spitting venom at her, and only my depleted energy holds me back from causing an even bigger scene. I am not even embarrassed. I am angry, and that anger feels good.

Another nurse, one I recognize, quickly appears and ushers the baffled nurse to the side. We are taken to a desk where the administrator takes our information. Another contraction starts. I grip the armrests and close my eyes in response. Jill comes in and immediately runs toward us. She places her hands on top of my shoulders, pressing down firmly and whispering, "You're on top of this."

A nurse takes us into an admitting room, not the same one we were in earlier, and shuts the door behind her. We wait through more agonizing rushes. I ask for pain relief, whatever they can give me. I'd planned on having an unmedicated birth, but at home I changed my mind and decided I wanted it all. "Anything you want," Aaron said.

They wheel in some sorry-looking nitrous oxide with a broken hose. I try it for a few contractions and give up. It doesn't do anything for the pain and it only restricts my breathing, which is strained and quick. Jill puts the TENS machine on me—its electrical pulses are meant to help me cope with the contractions—but it doesn't have time to work. I'm already in full-blown labor.

Then she tells me, "I am going to take some pictures for you and Aaron." I look at her quizzically, wondering why we would want pictures of any of this. "You don't ever have to look at them," she continues. "But just in case you want them one day, I'll keep them in a safe place for you."

"Alright," I say. I don't understand, but I trust her.

I request an epidural, as soon as possible. The exhaustion, the emotional toll, the physical pain, the mental agony—they are all at levels beyond what I can handle. If I'm going to finish this, I need just a few minutes to regain an ounce of strength.

Our midwife, Susie, arrives around midnight. She exhales audibly as she steps into the room. Her hair is braided down her back, with small wisps escaping at the nape of her neck. She gathers gloves and gauze and tools from a tray, the crystal bracelets stacked up on her wrists rattling as she works.

"Susie has lost a son too," Jill says.

"Really?" I gaze at her desperately, and she nods. I can almost sense her ache. I wonder if this kind of pain will be obvious to me now, a secret language spoken among a secret club of the bereaved. Learning that she knows the pain I am feeling, I feel instantly heartbroken and grateful at the same time. There she is, still living, still moving, still delivering babies even. Somehow, she is surviving. Maybe I will too.

Susie asks if she can perform a cervical check. She talks me through each step, gently preparing me for the discomfort. "You're seven centimeters," she announces. "I don't imagine it'll be long now." She smiles kindly and hurries out the door to speed up our admitting.

Later, I will learn that the nurses originally booked us into one of the smaller rooms in the windowless birthing suites on the first floor, the ones with paper-thin walls that let in the cries of mothers and babes from the other rooms on all sides. Jill and Susie advocated to move us upstairs, where the rooms are new and spacious and beautifully renovated, with windows looking out to courtyards. Upstairs, we don't have to see or hear what we'd longed to experience ourselves. Not much can make our situation better, but that small act certainly does. At least our birth will be our own.

At one thirty the anesthesiologist comes in to administer my epidural. He is young, another resident, but he is calm and confident. I start to relax, a little. I'm already fully dilated and can feel the pressure of the baby's head, but if I have just a few minutes to breathe, everything will be alright. The anesthesiologist numbs a patch on my spine, inserts the epidural catheter, and starts the drip. The cool rush of fluid passes through the tubes over my shoulder and I breathe through the next few contractions. As they start to slow down, I catch my breath. I bring myself back into the room and notice it is unexpectedly calm. Our midwife, our doula, and the labor nurse surround us, steadily going about their jobs. No fussing, no panic, no rush. There is peace—one I imagine could be attributed to God. It's strange to say, but suddenly the birth feels like the one I've been imagining. It feels beautiful.

My waters break in a dramatic gush shortly after the epidural. With one quick check Susie quietly says that it's time to start pushing, if I'm ready. I look to Aaron and have to blink away the tears. This is it. We are about to bring our son into the world and then, too quickly, say goodbye. I look at the clock—it's 2:00 AM on our due date—and grip Aaron's hand as I nod. I start to breathe our baby down and out, fully aware of every movement despite the epidural, as I gently push through each contraction.

"Remember to smile," Aaron whispers in my ear.

I forget myself for a moment and laugh as I bear down. He squeezes my hand and smiles with me. We'd been told in prenatal classes that smiling during the pushing stage could help minimize tearing. There's no longer a need to worry for the health of our baby, so he directs his worries to me. That he remembers this and voices it is a tremendous act of love.

Jill keeps assuring me that I'm doing an incredible job. She tells me my body is made for this, encourages me by saying that everything is stretching well. Then finally, a few pushes later, relief. I take our baby from Susie's hands and pull him up onto my chest. Aaron cuts the umbilical cord. At 2:24 AM on April 4, 2015, our beautiful son is born, still.

● ☾ ●

IN THE IMMEDIATE moments after his birth, we pore over every flawless inch of his strong body. He is the perfect mixture of us both. I see Aaron's nose, head shape, and long fingers and toes—he would have been tall. But he has my eyes, dimpled chin, and shock of black hair. I don't believe it's bias when I think that he's a striking baby. These moments are both the happiest and the most painful I've ever known. There will never be enough of them.

Then Susie says the words we never thought we'd hear:

"We know what happened."

"You do?" Aaron asks.

"There's a tight true knot in his umbilical cord," she replies. This knot is what killed him. Jill shows me a photo on her camera, zooming in on the center. The cord is dark and rich with life-sustaining fluids on one side of the knot, and on the other side, the one closest to his body, it is pale. Nothing was getting through. He was starved of all that was created to provide for him.

I don't ask to see the real thing. It doesn't occur to me that I might need to hold the knot that took the life from my own flesh and blood. Later, I will think I would have appreciated knowing how that felt.

True knots are rare, happening in about 1.2 percent of all pregnancies. And even more rarely are they fatal, because usually the knot doesn't tighten so severely.[1] We are told he must have done a few somersaults and tied it when he was very small—it was so close to his body. Then when he dropped in preparation for his birth, it would have tightened—slowly or quickly, we'll never know.

My heart is heavy knowing what happened. On one hand, it's a small relief to know it wasn't something we did or didn't do: ultrasounds can find knots, but because they are so rare, they aren't routinely screened for, so often go undetected. But that same knowledge brings tremendous grief; his passing happened completely out of our control. We couldn't have protected him from this.

Our labor nurse, Rose, looks at him lying on my chest. "He's perfect," she says. "Does he have a name?"

"Reid."

We decided months ago. We started referring to him by name in the third trimester, even though we kept Theo as a backup. But Reid fits him—a tribute to my maternal grand-father, Patrick Reid. Parents, siblings, and friends all used it, near the end. We knew who he was meant to be.

Aaron calls both of our parents: "He's here." Less than an hour after his birth, my parents arrive. I watch with pride as they lay eyes on him for the first time, gushing over how per-fect he is and commenting on which of us he looks like and why. Then I fall apart as they too mourn the loss of a life they have held close to their hearts. It dawns on me that though he died before anyone got to know him, he still made an impact, is still loved, and that many are grieving his death. We are not alone in this loss.

Time passes; nurses come and go. My wet sheets are changed out for fresh ones; I'm given a new hospital gown.

Aaron sleeps now on the couch next to my bed, and my parents doze in the corner by the window. It's still dark out, and the room is quiet. I lie with Reid in my arms. When I close my eyes, I can so easily pretend that he is just sleeping too, that any second he'll wiggle the way he did in my belly, or cry out to be fed. I memorize the weight of his body in my arms, imprint the image of his face in my mind.

I'm not an early-morning person. I'm not even a daylight person. That's not to say I'm not ambitious, but days often slip away from me. I can probably count the number of sunrises I've seen on both hands. They're sleepy and cold and pass too quickly. I'm a sunset child. A creature of the night, who thrives on the light from the moon and the stars. My best work is done past midnight. For me, three AM is bedtime, not rise-and-shine time.

The moments before the sun appears can take your breath away. Adventures of the night. The wine-filled evenings with secrets that linger in the air. Those times you went skinny-dipping. That night those sparklers singed your hair. The dreams you lived in before they escaped into the morning sky. The birth of your first child.

In these hours while the dark endures, I hold on to the time that the black skies give me, illuminated only by the stars and the lingering effect of the full blood moon of the eclipse. Until sunrise, Reid is heavy in my arms and perfect in his body. With family surrounding us, and without the reality of the light, I can almost imagine everything is as we've dreamed it would be. And in many unexpected ways, it is.

When the sun comes up, the clock will start ticking. We are on borrowed time; Reid has already started to change. But for this moment, in the magic of the night, he is safe in my arms, protected from the harshness of light and time. Reid is simply my baby who has just been born.

4

IT IS STILL early morning, but through the window the darkness is softening. Aaron is holding Reid on the make shift bed beside mine. My parents have stepped out of the room to give us some privacy as our nurse, Rose, does an assessment. She checks my blood pressure first, then massages my uterus to help it contract. As she turns the soft flesh of my empty belly into dough beneath her knuckles, I hear a loud gush of liquid.

"Oh!" she exclaims. She lifts up the sheet to examine what has come out of me and with relief assures me it is just urine. "Do you need to pee?" she asks.

I have to think about it for a moment. "I don't know," I say. She looks at me, clearly confused, then checks a screen over my shoulder. It is then that she realizes that the epidural drip has been left running. She mutters a few words under her breath. I say a dozen tiny prayers of gratitude that someone else's oversight gave me a few more hours free of physical pain.

Rose helps me over to the bathroom and places a basin over the toilet bowl. "You won't quite know how to do this because you're still so numb. But it's mind over matter," she counsels me. I ask her to run the water, but before she turns the tap my body knows what it needs to do.

Back in bed, I'm overcome with fatigue. Rose asks if we'd like to give Reid a bath. I tell Aaron he can if he wants to; I'm just going to close my eyes for a minute or two. Aaron, looking every bit as tired as I feel, asks Rose if she can do it instead.

"Of course," she says. She grabs a yellow plastic cup, a basin, and a travel-sized bottle of Johnson's baby shampoo and sets up the bath on the counter across the room from us.

I peer over to her every now and then, watching her carefully rub the soap into Reid's hair as I drift in and out of half sleep. Later, I will read that it is a ritual in many cultures to cleanse the body of the deceased after they have passed—it's part of the mourning process. We are only doing what is expected after birth, trying to grasp at any sense of normalcy that we can. But I am glad that he is being cared for this way.

When she is finished, she brings him back over to me. I hold him against my chest and breathe him in.

"Do you want to dress him?" Susie asks, coming back into the room.

We put him in the newborn outfit I'd packed long ago to bring him home in. A white and gray outfit with mittens and a hat and a tiny sweater to match. I struggle to get the onesie over his head—I've never dressed a baby before. Susie comes over and holds Reid's head in place as I pull the fabric down over his face. I study it then, the way it is different from other newborn faces I've seen, the way it is changing still.

It feels strange to be able to do these things: weigh and bathe and dress him. As he lies on my lap, it occurs to me that he was a part of me for his whole entire life and now here he is, suddenly separate. I want to repair our bond, to somehow absorb him. I want to find our way back to the time and place where he was alive. I want to be together again.

I always thought, somehow, that death would follow the rules. This was supposed to be a beginning; now we are at an end. In this world we now live in, life-altering things happen with no apparent reason or warning.

The rest of our family members arrive. Aaron's parents, our sisters and their significant others, my maternal grandmother. They enter our room one by one, and it is torture to look them in the eye. I am keenly aware that had Reid been safely delivered into our arms, this is exactly the scene that would have played out—family and friends gathering at our bedside, only it would have been to welcome our son into the world with celebration. Now, as I realize with my stomach churning, they are coming to us in sorrow. It isn't fair. And yet seeing Reid in the arms of our loved ones feels right. I only wish more people could be here to hold him.

I watch Aaron hold our son, both pain and pride written on his face, a father's love for his child bursting into the room. I don't ever want to forget this moment. My own heart throbs to see how Reid can't meet his gaze, to grasp that he will never get the opportunity. I think of the God that I thought I believed in and can't understand why we find ourselves in this reality. Still, I find some comfort in knowing that the first face Reid saw was His.

I am sure I only close my eyes again for a minute, but now everyone else is gone and a woman I don't recognize is at my bedside. The skies are starting to brighten and I know that things will start to move quickly now. The woman introduces herself as the social worker and starts to talk about support groups, funeral arrangements, forms to fill out. I can't absorb any of it. Reid is still in my arms, wrapped in the swaddle I had packed in his hospital bag months ago. A white swaddle with red, gray, and black details, speckled with bears—I'd forgotten how cute the pattern was. I adjust his body; the weight of him is making my hand go numb. He is right here, in my arms, and this woman is talking about all of these terrible things we'll have to do when he is "gone." *Gone.* I mull that over and continue to nod as she speaks. I don't care what she is saying; everything she is saying feels wrong anyway. I continue to stare at my beautiful boy as she talks.

"…you won't get a birth certificate," I hear her say. "So, here's the form for the certificate of remembrance that you can get. It's a really beautiful memento; they do an excellent job." She taps her pen lightly to her clipboard as if to emphasize that point.

My eyes jump up to meet hers. "Sorry, what did you just say?" I can hear my voice crack as my mind fumbles to process her words.

"I'm… I'm so sorry," she falters. "You don't get a birth certificate."

"We don't get a birth certificate?" This woman can't be serious. "But he was born five hours ago. Look at him."

"I know. I'm so sorry. So sorry. But he didn't take a breath. So..." she trails off and gives me a pitiful half smile as she looks at my son. "He's perfect."

"Yes," is all I can manage as I choke back the tears, "he's perfect."

I wrestle with many things immediately following Reid's death, but none more than this: What happens when the order of birth and death are disrupted? Stillbirth goes against the way most people think about life and death, and the timeline in which they occur. It's unsettling.

When death takes a life before birth, is it a life? I don't know. I don't think there will ever be an answer that feels certain, or one that is right for everyone. But right here, right now, I wonder, is it really just a single breath of air that creates a life? And the absence of it that makes a death?

The person down the hall from me with a breathing baby to hold will receive a paper, one that confirms that, yes, a birth has taken place. I, however, am only given permission to remember. No proof of birth. No proof of either life or death. It doesn't make sense that someone in government, someone who doesn't know me, whom I've never met, has the power to decide what this baby means to our family. Nothing makes sense. He is right here in my arms.

At seven thirty, our new day nurse, Ava, comes in to introduce herself. I like her immediately. She is young, but it's clear that all she wants to do is make the hours we have left with Reid special. She says she will call a photographer to take portraits, if we want. She also says the hospital chaplain will be arriving soon and she can ask him to do a baptism. Whatever we want, she will make it happen. She repeats this to us over and over again.

The problem is, we don't know what we want. None of my lists or plans included things we might want to do with our stillborn son while we have the chance.

"We should do everything we can, right?" I ask Aaron.

"I think so," he agrees. "We won't get another opportunity."

So we do what we can. We say yes to the professional portraits and the Christian baptism and the castings of his hands and feet. We do it all. And yet, we know we will always wish we'd done more.

The longer I hold him, the more he changes. Fluids escape through his nose from somewhere else in his body, like a river carving new forks in its passage. I wipe the liquid up with the edges of his swaddle, and for a moment I imagine that he just has a runny nose.

Right then, Micaela, one of my closest friends, who is also a nurse in the Pediatric Intensive Care Unit at the children's hospital down the hall, appears. She is balancing a large, flat rectangle, covered in pale-green hospital blankets, in her outstretched hands. She is crying.

"We have to put him on ice now," she chokes out. Only then do I notice the rectangle in her arms is a bed of ice. "But he'll still be warm. We'll wrap him up in this." She tucks the swaddle up under his chin. I look at her and help with the swaddle. Should I tell her that he won't be warm? Should I tell her it doesn't matter? Reid isn't in his body anymore. This is a corpse.

They say that some families take the body home. Sometimes it helps to see the child in the car seat, the nursery, the bassinet. I almost believe that I can. I'll strap Reid in and we'll walk through the halls toward the elevator; another new family will lean over to marvel at the tiny being we too are bringing home. Then their faces will melt with horror. "Yes, well, he died," we'll say. "But isn't he perfect?"

No, no. There is absolutely no way I could manage it. I am glad they offered, though. Later, it will be the things they didn't offer—things I didn't know I could have done—that I will grow to regret: not taking a lock of his hair or looking at his eyes or singing songs to him, not taking every opportunity to make more memories with him as a family. But if I bring him home I'll have to bring him back, and I don't imagine I'll have the willpower to do it. They will have to send someone to pry his cold body out of my trembling hands. "But isn't he perfect?"

At four thirty in the afternoon, after fourteen hours and six minutes with Reid, Aaron and I look at each other. Our eyes are swollen and red. I've never seen such a look of defeat on his face. We haven't been given a limit to the time we can spend with our son, but in this moment we know, as well as we will ever know, that we are ready to leave his body. As much as I don't want to say goodbye, I also desperately need to.

"Are you ready?" I ask, knowing how stupid the question sounds. He nods, knowing how wrong the answer feels.

Earlier, Ava had offered to be with Reid after we left, so we buzz her now, ask her to come into the room. "We think it's time. Could you look after him? Could you hold him for us?" we whisper into the bedside monitor.

A crackle, and then: "Of course. I'll be right there."

She enters the room minutes later and stands to the side, interlacing her hands, then letting them hang at her hips. She waits. Aaron collects our bags from in front of the bed. Then he bends down and kisses the smooth skin of Reid's forehead. I reach my hands underneath the cotton of his clothing, picking him up off the bed of ice. A chill travels through my body. I draw him up to my chest. Slowly, I press him into me and take a deep breath, soaking up as much of him as I can. And then—and then I place him in Ava's arms and walk toward the door.

As I cross the threshold I look back. All around us these guttural cries are ringing. I don't realize that they are coming from me.

"You can come back," Ava says, wiping tears from beneath the thick black frames of her glasses. "You can come back."

I walk back in and give Reid one last kiss. My fingers linger on his chest, where his arms are delicately crossed. I turn to leave, but my arm refuses to follow. His hand, soft and limp in my grasp, slides gently toward the floor. His hat has fallen a little off his head, and his black hair is visible at the edge. His lips are a deep, blood red. I glance at the clock above the hospital bed. 4:45 PM. And then I turn my back and walk away. This time, I don't—I can't—look back.

● ☾ ●

WE ARE FINALLY alone. The echo in our apartment seems amplified in the absence of the noise that should have filled it on our return from the hospital. I look around at all the evidence of our plans. The infant tub on the back of the door, the room stacked ceiling-high with baby gear, the pregnancy books scattered across tables. Then the magnet with the paging details on it, sitting right where we left it on the coffee table.

I close my eyes and whisper to Aaron, "I need to shower, but I need help." He holds me as we shuffle toward the bathroom. He supports me under my arms and lowers me down on the toilet. He undresses me, slowly. As my shirt brushes past my face I catch a scent that is both foreign and familiar to me. It is the scent of *him*—of his birth.

In Dr. Patrick O'Malley's book *Getting Grief Right*, I'll later read about a similar experience he had upon sensing something that reminded him of his infant son who'd passed. As a psychotherapist, he researched all aspects of his grief, and wrote:

> *That innocent sensory stimulus had cut straight to the place in my brain where the memories and feelings of Ryan would be forever stood. It is called the* limbic system, *a primitive part of our brain where human emotions are believed to be centered. A sight or smell might register there and is then interpreted and named by more advanced parts of our cognitive apparatus. The pungent aroma of antiseptic soap produced tears, which my brain could eventually link to the hospital.*

At first, I notice the Ivory Snow. I recall the days I sat in his nursery with his hand-washed outfits in my lap. The smell of the detergent would travel on the breeze coming in through the corner window and I'd close my eyes, basking in it. Even though he only wore one outfit, I know that smell will probably always tie me to his life. It will always remind me of the days I spent washing his things and organizing his drawers.

Then I notice the Johnson's baby shampoo that Rose washed his hair with. I summon the hazy memories of her lathering his head with bubbles and gently rinsing them out with water that spilled from the yellow plastic cup.

And another scent, one I can't recognize, one I can only assume is death. I inhale deeply, bringing my hands up toward my nose, as close as I can. "I still smell like him," I whisper to Aaron.

"Me too," he whispers back.

A single tear rolls down my cheek. I don't want to wash it off. I don't want to be one step closer to reaching our first day without Reid. I don't want any of it. The minute I enter that shower it will all be gone. The beginning of erasing what little proof I have of his existence.

Once in bed, I look at the packets of sleeping pills beside me. They have given me enough to put me into a deep, medically induced sleep, nothing more. I punch two out into my palm and stroke their shiny blue surface before placing them on the tip of my tongue.

I wait for sleep to come, but it never does. My insomnia is as much biological as situational. I am supposed to be up all night with a baby depending on me for survival. I know that he has died. But my body doesn't.

In the morning, Susie comes over. I am still in bed, the covers drawn up underneath my chin. She sits next to me and talks about the birth, discussing the stiches and some of the changes my body is going through. I ask her to tell me about her son, the one who died, and listen closely as she does. When it is time for her to leave she hands me a brown paper bag, crumpled at the top to keep whatever it is holding contained. "You'll want to wash these," she says.

I peer inside. Neatly folded at the bottom are Reid's clothes. I sigh, "Oh." I roll the top down again and thank her.

I don't know why, but I assumed he would be cremated in them. Or at the very least make it to the funeral home wearing them. All I can picture is that somewhere in the basement of the hospital he is lying naked on a cold metal tray, sealed in a bag and completely alone. Someone would have been tasked with undressing him. I cringe at the thought of him being handled by strangers.

After Susie leaves, when I can allow myself to surrender to the pain, I take his clothes out of the bag and gently lay them on my lap. They smell sour and are stained through with blood. Then, at the very bottom of the bag, I find the small bracelet with a metal heart that I'd been allowed to tie to his wrist. I have the matching necklace, a heart with its middle punched out—the middle that makes up his pendant—sitting on my bedside table. It is meant so that the griever can always feel close to the one they grieve. They can look at the hole in the heart and imagine it tethered to their loved one, as it was when they left them. But here it is in my hands. I throw the bag with the bracelet against the wall and scream into my pillow. Someone lied. Or someone made a mistake, placed it in the bag of his belongings instead of tossing it in the trash and letting us continue to believe that it remains with him. I'm not sure which of the two options feels worse.

The midwives pay their official visits and then many more, bringing their love and grief with them as they enter our apartment. Fiona, the midwife who cared for us during our pregnancy, visits this afternoon. She was out of town when Reid was born. The team called her while she was on vacation to let her know and she broke down. "But her pregnancy was perfect!" she sobbed. "And they're so young!"

When she arrives at our door she is already red-faced from crying. I can't imagine how difficult it must be for her to step into our pain, to have cared for us as she did and then have this be the outcome. I wonder if she thought we'd blame her. She could have easily never come and we wouldn't have faulted her for that. But the fact that she does means the world to us.

Fiona says that she was there when they told the other couples in our prenatal group, that they all send their condolences and their love. She says that one of the fathers was so upset he had to leave the room. It relieves me to hear this—not because the father had hurt, but because his act of mourning somehow acknowledges our grief in a way I need.

● ☾ ●

IN THE FIRST days after, my mind is at war with itself. I want to remember it all. In photos, diaries, and old texts from when I was pregnant. I ask Jill for the pictures from Reid's birth, lose myself in the tears and longing they bring. I also want the days to fade into oblivion, to wipe the pain from my memory. But I can't figure out how to keep Reid alive in my heart without the ache. Will it always be like this? I have to believe it will get better. But then, do I want it to? Because when it gets better, what will be lost in the process? Already, I know that it will come at a price.

Aaron and I binge-watch *Mad Men*. We sit on the couch for hours, only rising to make tea and refill our bowls with cereal—our fridge is full of homemade meals, but we can't stomach any of them. We think TV will be safe because babies never die there. But we quickly learn that nothing is safe anymore.

In one episode, Don Draper and his creative team are about to pitch a major idea to land the advertising for American Airlines. But on Good Friday, of all days, they get the news that their contact at the airline has been fired. Don is exasperated; the team is in a panic. Then someone asks what it means for them and Don says, "Now we have to deliver a stillborn baby."

We press pause instantly and stare at the screen.

"Did you just hear that?" Aaron asks.

"Did that really just happen?" I can't believe it. We rewind and watch it again to be sure we aren't losing our minds. Before Reid died, I'd never thought about stillbirth—it wasn't a word I could ever recall hearing. Suddenly, it seems to be everywhere.

But that particular line of Don's sticks with me, and I think a lot about what the writers meant to say with it. The idea was still beautiful, that much was clear. Fully formed, perfect. But it would never live on as intended. Regardless, they had to go through the motions, as they would with any other pitch. And, I think, as a mother would with any other baby.

My milk appears on the Tuesday. My breasts are hot and engorged, vessels full of liquid gold with nowhere to go. One of the first things I asked about after Reid was born was whether or not my milk would still come in. I thought that my body would understand there wasn't a baby to feed, so I was surprised, and devastated, to learn that the answer was yes. I was told how to help it dry up, and my hand was held as I cried about needing that advice.

I am hit with a fresh wave of grief when my milk does come in. Knowing that it will disappear without being used is overwhelming. Later I will find out—and wish that I knew earlier—that I could have donated Reid's milk to a baby in need, given purpose to my days. For a little while at least, I think I might have liked that milk to nourish a life, instead of slowly drying up and taking the last physical connection I had to my son with it.

I sit on the couch with frozen cabbage leaves on my breasts, with holes cut out in the center of them for the nipples. Soon, everything I own reeks of cabbage. My bras, my shirts, my sheets. Even my body—it seems to be seeping out of my pores. The smell is worse than the pain, somehow, so I get rid of the cabbage. Instead, I drink gallons of peppermint and sage tea. I make cold compresses from facecloths drenched in ice water with peppermint oil sprinkled on top and soak in baths scented with the essential oils. Sometimes globs of the oil pool together and land undiluted on my skin, burning red patches into my flesh, and I relish the feeling. Some other, separate pain I can pour my own into.

Really, I just miss him. That's it. That's the whole problem. I miss him every single second. My body cries for him. In tears, blood, and milk it wails deep into the burden of the night. And there is nothing that can soothe me dry.

● ☽ ●

IT'S FRIDAY, APRIL 10, one week *after*, the first of what I assume will be many terrible anniversaries. I wake up often during the night, unable to sleep knowing that one week earlier, in those very hours, Reid had passed away inside of me. *I had slept through it.* But the date has another significance, too. I know that today, one of my closest friends will be having her baby.

Amy lives in Ottawa, but we'd become friends at university years earlier, when she was the resident assistant of my dorm. We bonded instantly over our love of books and organization and handwritten cards. She had a single room and we would often end up there, staying up late as we talked into the night, sipping hot tea from the cafeteria, me lying on the floor and her propped up on her side in her bed. After I told her I was pregnant with Reid, she'd FaceTimed me—just to congratulate me, I'd thought at first. She had inquired about what fruit size Reid was at the time. A peach, I'd said, thinking her question was odd. But then she asked, "Do you think your peach might like to play with our blueberry?" and held her own ultrasound image up to the screen.

When Amy was twenty weeks pregnant, she was diagnosed with vasa previa, a rare condition where the connection of the umbilical cord to the placenta crosses over the opening of the cervix. Her waters breaking suddenly would mean a very real risk of both Amy and her child dying. At thirty-two weeks, she was moved into the hospital and put on bed rest. At thirty-six weeks, she was scheduled to have a cesarean.

I wake up braced for news about her delivery. It embarrasses me to admit it, but I was never really worried about her or her baby before Reid's passing. Whenever she called me from the hospital during those last weeks of pregnancy, fearing what might happen, I hardly listened. I simply promised her that everything would be okay. It wasn't that I knew the outcome; it was that I resisted the possibility of a different one. Because bad things didn't happen to people I knew. And they didn't happen to me. Now, all I expect is bad news.

Instead, when I grab my phone, there is a text from Brittany announcing that her daughter, Charlotte, has been born safely. She tells me she is experiencing all the expected emotions: happiness, relief, and love. She also feels deep sorrow, grief, and heartbreak. Joy because her daughter is here, but anguish because I didn't get that same moment. After we shared everything during our pregnancies, including near-identical due dates, she can't believe that we aren't sharing the same outcome. I am grateful for her honesty and happy for her, and also so incredibly broken.

Amy's announcement comes later that morning. They'd been waiting to find out the sex, and she tells me they have a daughter, Grace. The delivery went well. Grace is in the NICU to help with her breathing, but Amy assures me she will be okay. Amy will be okay too.

Although I know better than to make assumptions based on the sex of a baby, that both Amy and Brittany had daughters is a consolation to me, one that could lead to a gentler kind of grief as they grow and Reid doesn't. I imagine their homes filling with the things little girls sometimes like, and it might be a little less obvious exactly what I'm missing.

Finally, I fall into my first deep sleep that afternoon, collapsing on the couch out of relief and pure exhaustion. I've survived the first anniversary. I've survived the births of my friends' babies. Now to survive the rest.

5

THE FIRST DEATH I remember was when a close friend of my parents, Miranda, passed away from breast cancer when I was fourteen. She worked for my father and was often around our home—she even nearly married my uncle Mike, once upon a time. She was alluring, with her slim frame and hair as dark as midnight. She was quite possibly one of the most beautiful women I'd ever seen. More than that, she had a calm presence that was only enhanced by her soothing voice—I still remember the sound of it all these years later.

I don't really remember much from when she was sick, just one time when I went out for a fancy lunch with her and my mom and she talked about all the fun wigs she got to wear. What I remember most about that lunch was the way she spoke about snowboarding. She talked about how much she loved it, and her eyes lit up when she did, and then she turned to me and told me she wanted to teach me someday. But we never got that chance. She died shortly after, and instead of my first snowboarding lesson I went to my first funeral.

Only it wasn't really a funeral. I asked my mom why everyone was in bright colors, smiling and crying and telling stories about her—it wasn't anything like what I'd seen in movies. She told me that Miranda wanted a celebration of life; she wanted those who knew her to remember and celebrate her for how she lived, not grieve for how she died. That stuck with me. At Miranda's party I decided I didn't want a funeral either when I died, though I didn't even know what a traditional funeral was like. And it's why we decide not to have one for Reid. I want to have a chance to celebrate him too.

Over the following week, I pour all my time and energy into working on Reid's baby album. I started it a month ago, figuring I wouldn't have time to add all the details from the pregnancy after he was born. I couldn't have known then that his firsts would also be his lasts: his first photo, first outfit, first diaper, first bath. His first cuddles with Mom and Dad. I change the wording throughout the book, making firsts into lasts or onlys, and fill the empty pages with pictures and writing. When it is finally done, I am devastated: the summary of his life fits into a single book, completed in only a few days.

I also include the story of his birth, which I have written and printed out. I started to write it the day after it happened, just to process exactly what it was that had happened, to get the facts down on paper, keep the timeline straight. But as I kept writing, all the feelings came back to me, again and again and again. The words became expression, the expression became a story, and through that story I felt the very beginnings of something I wouldn't dare yet call healing.

On the second Sunday after Reid's death, our family comes over to our apartment for the celebration of his life. Our home seems like the only appropriate place to have it. It is where his soul entered this world, and where it left it. These walls framed the span of his existence.

Everyone who has been a major part of Reid's life is here: our parents, our siblings and their significant others, a few friends, and my maternal grandparents. Aaron's brothers, Derek and Levi, flew in earlier in the week. Derek, who is just shy of two years younger than Aaron, has grown his beard long and pierced his ears through with wooden spikes while he was away. I notice that he has also taken to wearing baggy linen clothes. These are all things I would usually tease him about, but I don't have the heart to today. Or maybe my heart toward these things has softened—it seems cruel to judge anything so personal. Levi, Aaron's youngest brother, is the same age as Rebecca, who is five years younger than me. A few years back we entertained the idea of setting them up together, encouraging them to exchange school photos with little messages on the back. Now Levi attends school in Ontario, studying mathematics at the same small Christian university Derek had attended.

We gather in our living room and pass around the baby album. I watch our family as they look through the photos, reliving all the memories with him, and, finally, reading what I've written of his birth. I see them leaning in and out of their own pain as they read the story, just as I did while writing it.

They have every right to mourn, each of them being intimately connected to our loss, but maybe they needed this to give them permission.

After everyone has a chance to go through the album we reminisce about the pregnancy, about all the memories created during those nine months. There is talk about the first time we heard his glorious heartbeat at twelve weeks. About how I felt his kicks early, at sixteen weeks, and how even Aaron was able to feel them soon after.

As the conversation moves to the details of parties held for Reid and trips with family and the dreams they had of a future with him, I mostly remain quiet. I fear that if I open my mouth, it won't be words that come out but instead the awful, torturous sounds of grief. So I stay in one spot and drink peppermint tea and take in this community act of remembering. And I silently reflect on the wiggly companion who kept me company every hour of every day, who rolled when I ate sour foods and kicked his feet into my ribs as I walked. It was all so good, and all so short.

Then everyone writes down the questions that are in their hearts about Reid's passing, all the hows and whys. Or, if they feel called to, a letter for him instead. We seal them all in an envelope, which we will later take to the funeral home to be placed with Reid inside his casket. It was Aaron's idea. One more thing he can do for his son.

At the end of the day, Aaron speaks. "Nine months ago our lives changed," he begins, pausing to clear his throat. No parent should have to talk like this about their child. "I still remember the day I found out that Emma was pregnant. I was enjoying the sun in the lineup at the ferry terminal when my phone began to ring. This question was hanging over our heads so I was expecting the call, but when I saw her name my stomach began to do flips all the same."

The room is full of smiles as each person remembers the time we recounted this story to them. Aaron smiles too, and then continues. "Our nerves were soon replaced by excitement as we dreamed up questions and thought of all the plans we needed to make. That was truly the start of the lives that Emma and I felt we were meant to live."

I think of how true that is, of how quickly our motivation for everything became to create the best life we could for Reid. I reach for his hand and give it a little squeeze, and he squeezes back.

"Reid was intent on making himself known. He was energetic and mischievous. As he grew into his home, he learned how to hiccup regularly, preparing his lungs for the outside world. He discovered that when he had a little extra energy to burn, there was a lovely rib-shaped leg press that would provide him with the necessary resistance. He also loved to interact with the outside world, pushing back at me when I tickled his heels. As he grew, he was able to share more of himself with us, and I hope that he was able to learn about us in return."

I start to cry now. Because this is all we can talk about, this is all we'll ever know of him. And I want it all back. It is enough and he is our child and I want more of him.

"It feels like an injustice that we should learn so much about him, but never truly get the chance to meet him, to look into his eyes." He says what I am feeling, and I exhale in relief that he is feeling these things too. "What questions we had about our future together have been replaced with darker ones; our joy has turned to pain. We are grateful for the time that we were able to spend with him, but we wish we had more. More time to love him, more time to know him, like—" he falters now, struggling to make it through.

"What color were his eyes? What would his voice sound like? Would he be tall? What would he love to do? Was he shy or outgoing?" I look around the room and take in the wet faces and nodding heads, the evident grief of the group of family and friends who knew Reid best.

"These questions are tough ones to ask, but they are important. For though we will never find the answers, they will help us to remember him." He turns to me now, and his expression seems to tell me that this is a promise. "Remembering will keep him alive in our hearts."

A cry escapes my ninety-year-old grandfather, Reid's namesake. I've never seen him cry before, and seeing his tears—well, I think it says everything I cannot.

● ☾ ●

I WAKE THE next morning and change another pad, let the reminder that blood on bleached cotton brings sink in. I am a mother recovering from birth as much as I am a mother grieving the death of her child, and I often forget this. As I wash my hands, I let myself look up, slowly arriving to meet my gaze in the mirror for the first time since Reid died. My face appears both sunken from sorrow and swollen from a combination of tears and shifting hormones. My eyes seem to say they've seen too much sadness, and will now permanently rest in this pained state. My lips are neutral, and it's as if they're letting me know they're willing to continue on if I am.

I notice that despite the agony my physical body is in, emotionally I feel lighter today. Something in the marking of Reid's life, and the ritual of celebrating it, has released a bit of the burden I've been carrying. I decide to publish Reid's birth story on my blog. I documented and shared most other aspects of my pregnancy with my readers, and I don't see why I shouldn't share this too. I want others to know of Reid, and I want his life—and our grief—to be acknowledged. I want to be honest. And maybe my words can help one other person feel a little less alone.

I enter the title into the template, *Born Still but Still Born,* and take a deep breath. I have never written anything so personal before. Or so painful. But as I tell my story, creating some order out of the chaos in my mind, I begin to feel different—better, almost. The words can't change my reality—though I want them to—but they help me transform the unimaginable into something I can see. What I've written is a birth story, because Reid was still born. And I know it's a story I need to share.

I hit "publish" and wait, clutching my phone in my hand.

Within minutes, the comments start to roll in. Heartfelt condolences, which I expected, but they are still so powerful. I read their words:

Reid will live on because you gave him life. Thank you for being so brave...

I am so sorry Reid is not here, where he belongs...

I am truly sorry for your loss. May your memories of holding your boy in your arms sustain you in your grief.

And then the stories start coming. Within the first few hours, tens, then hundreds. Eventually there will be thousands of stories from those who have lost children. Their names proudly written out, next to a date, on my blog. So many of them stillborn, more than I ever anticipated. They write:

My first son was stillborn at full term on August 8, 2008...

I felt as if you were telling my story as I read this. Instead of juice, I was eating watermelon and cupcakes trying to will my baby to move inside of me. Instead of watching Friends, *we came home from the hospital and had a campfire in the back yard...*

My heart breaks for you both. A good friend of mine recently delivered her sleeping baby.

A few days later Aaron wakes me up to say that Reid's story has gone viral. Earlier, we had watched Google Analytics as the number of readers on my site had climbed from ten at a time to fifty. When I look at it now, the number is in the thousands. Over the next days our story is shared on American political pages with millions of followers, usually pro-life conservative groups. It appears in all of our local newspapers. Requests for media appearances and in-person interviews flood my inbox. The story spreads across the country. Soon after, it reaches countries all over the world.

At first, I'm hit with anxiety. I wrote about our personal experience because the words needed to come out. I didn't expect publicity. And I didn't want our story, or Reid's life, to be politicized. But because he died before his birth, he was suddenly being used as part of a narrative of pro-life versus pro-choice. I read harsh comments such as *It's a fetus, this mother should get over it,* next to imploring messages like *I wish every mother about to abort her child could read this.* In sharing what happened to me, I had no interest in taking sides in that debate—I don't think that it's either-or, all the time, no matter what. I am only pro-supporting-people-in-their-own-unique-situations, given their unique beliefs and circumstances. I wanted to tell our story, as it applies to us, with no intention of implying that everyone's feelings and views in similar experiences should be the same. I hope that this specific kind of attention will fade quickly.

At the same time, as I watch more and more people come to my blog to find Reid's story, a strange sense of peace spreads over me. All of these people are learning about our son. When a baby dies before they have a chance to create their own story, I think one of the biggest fears parents have is that they will disappear, be forgotten. It's up to those who knew them to spread their legacy, should that be something that's in their hearts to do. It strikes me that these people might never have heard Reid's name had he not died.

A few weeks before, when Reid passed away, I didn't know of a single person who had experienced a late-term stillbirth. All I could think of were the stories I'd come across in books or television. I think of the book *The Light Between Oceans* by M.L. Stedman, set in the 1920s, where the main characters experience two miscarriages and one stillbirth. I think of how a live baby washed up in a boat on that lone island they lived on, so soon after the stillbirth, how the wife, Isabel, took that baby to her breast, nursed her. I think of how her whole body would have been aching for the experience: the letdown, the relief from engorgement, the suckling child before her.

I think of the show *Call the Midwife*, set in the 1950s in East London, that I watched while I was pregnant; how I fast-forwarded though any scenes where the baby died because I believed those were problems of the past.

A part of me knew all along that there must be real-life stories that inspired these accounts, must be other people out there who have had losses like mine, who also felt isolated and unsure about what to do. I just had no idea how many there were. I wasn't prepared for my story to resonate with so many. I wasn't prepared for millions of people to read it, and then have many of them actually respond.

As I read each message that reaches me, devour their condolences and stories, I feel, somehow, that I am being validated. I left the hospital thinking that I must be the only person in the world this had happened to, that I'd done something terrible to invite it, that I couldn't grieve this loss—didn't know how. But here from my living room couch—handwritten cards piled high beside me and my computer screen open to the latest email—I see that none of that is true. It is a great privilege to receive their stories, and they are a gift to me. These words tell me that I am not alone, they assure me that I did not cause this, and they provide a road map to the kind of grief that once seemed so invisible.

I start to wonder if we can experience healing through our stories. We all have a story to tell, after all, and we all learn from other people's stories too. Even though these stories can't make our losses okay, is it possible they can bring meaning to our suffering? I am not the first person to have lost their child. And sadly, I will not be the last. Finding healing after such a thing, I think, shouldn't have to be lonely.

● ☾ ●

WE DECIDE TO have Reid's body cremated. The conversation is short, as both options seem awful. With a burial, I picture his body all alone and decaying below us with myself safe and warm at home, thinking only of the child lying in the cold, hard ground miles away. Or I imagine us moving one day, abandoning him in his grave. I do not want us to be separated.

So then it has to be cremation. Doesn't it? I see an image of him entering a tomb of flames, reduced to dust in an instant. It is horrible too, but it is the awful that we feel most at peace with. We can keep his ashes with us wherever life takes us next.

Later, I'll speak to a cremator about the cremation process. I will enter a sizeable room lit from above by florescent panels, its air filled with a steady, low hum. On the far-left side sits the machine, a large brick oven, that generates this noise. Directly in front of it, a broken fluorescent panel exposes two long naked bulbs.

I will see the casket, fashioned from particle board with words from loved ones scribbled in permanent marker all over the outside. It rests on top of a large metal platform, on a bed of metal rods that spin when one end of it is raised to help the casket glide into the kiln.

I will walk over to Gale, the cremator, and try to calculate if I can ask him what's been on my mind. I will look him in the eye and ask if the process for babies is any different than what I am witnessing. I will ask because I can't get the sound of the casket thudding into the base of the furnace chamber out of my mind. I can't imagine a casket a fraction of the size making it off that conveyor.

Gale will not falter. He will be calm and return my gaze before asking, "Approximately what size?"

"An infant," I will start to cry. "Around eight pounds."

I will be surprised to see Gale start to cry too, silent tears hitting his cheeks. He will respond with this: "I place babies in by hand. And instead of heating up the chamber first, I keep it cool. I think it's gentler that way. Most people in my profession do this too, and I can't speak for everyone, but I've learned that we all have the utmost respect for the soul and its journey." He will lift his glasses slightly to wipe underneath his eyes and adjust them back in place. "I like to go longer for babies too. So that I know for sure that it's done all at once."

I will thank him, because this is information I would rather know about than wonder.

The first weekend we were home from the hospital, I made a list of questions to ask the funeral home:

Where will he be cremated?

How long until we can get him back?

Will he be cremated on his own or with other babies?

I wrote down the last one after someone mentioned it on an online forum I found. She said that some funeral homes cremated babies together to make sure there were "enough" ashes to give the family. Apparently some babies are so small, she wrote, that there was practically nothing left of them.

When we walk through the doors of the funeral home, the middle-aged receptionist looks up. I notice her blouse has a snag in it near the neckline. I appreciate that; it seems almost a kind gesture to meet the grieving slightly unkempt.

"Hello," she says, pushing her glasses back up to the top of her nose. "Are you Reid's parents?"

We nod. She offers her condolences and leads us to a large conference room down the hall. I keep pressing the tip of my nail into the belly of my palm, focusing on the pain it causes. I will use this trick many times over the years that follow to keep tears at bay.

She tells us that our caseworker will be in shortly and gently places a binder on the table in front of the chair across from us. Before she stands up to go, she meets my gaze and pauses.

"I'm not supposed to show emotion or talk about anything personal with our families, but I can't *not* say anything. How can you not cry when something this awful happens? I read your blog, and I just need to say how sorry I am." Tears are pooling in the corners of her eyes and her mouth begins to tremble. She looks from me to Aaron and back to me again. I thank her for saying something, and her hands fiddle at her center for a short while before she finally rests a palm on top of my own. She strokes it once and gives it a pat and then she excuses herself and leaves us alone.

A few minutes later, the type of man you'd expect to work at a funeral home enters the room. His dark hair is gelled into a perfect comb-over and his suit is immaculately pressed, its gray fabric registering not a speck of lint.

"I am so sorry for your loss," he begins.

He sits down across from us and goes through the binder. Discussions of the crematorium and ceremonies are had, presumably—I don't register any of them. I do pay attention when he leads us into the room that holds all the urns. Countless vases and boxes and vials line the walls. And then, at the back, the single shelf that holds the ones small enough for infants.

After it all, we end up back at reception. The receptionist with the kind face prints out an invoice and reads it over before saying, "That will be $183.75." Tears begin to fill her eyes again.

I hand her my Visa. Not even two hundred dollars to reduce our son's body to ash. I don't know why, but I want it to be more.

● ☾ ●

MEMORIES HAUNT ME of our walk through the hospital halls with empty arms. I was lucky, in that I never heard babies crying during our stay. But I did hear their screams as we walked toward the parking lot, as quickly as my stretched body would allow us. I couldn't block out the sounds. I felt faint and dissociated, my legs threatening to collapse under me.

I keep coming back to one moment that I just can't release. We had turned the corner by the nurses' station when we walked by a new father, happily standing there, bouncing his healthy baby in his arms. The first baby I saw after leaving Reid. Mere hours after our family had been broken, I was witnessing the joy of a family that had just become whole. I wanted to feel that so badly.

My anger latches on to the memory and won't let go. I would have taken that father's happiness from him, if it meant I could know his joy. My rage surprises me, and fuels me, too. It's easier to be angry. I can't blame the midwives or the hospital staff or anyone else, so this father and child are as good as any other people to take the brunt of it. I'm not proud of myself, but I don't much care. Why did *they* get to bring their baby home?

Since sharing Reid's birth story, I continue to blog through my experience, and I decide not to hide anything I'm feeling. I share my aches, my doubts and fears, my most intimate thoughts. And the more I share them, the more people write in to share theirs. I'm amazed at how my vulnerability is being embraced with more vulnerability—that others are not only willing to see me in my pain, but to meet me in it too.

Then one day, as I'm reading through emails, one message stops me cold. I read through the words, letting the guilt and shame wash over me.

You don't know me, but I saw your tears on April 4. My daughter was born at 5:00 PM (on the dot) on Good Friday.

The next day, I took her for her first walk out of the room to get more sunlight. I was particularly grateful right at that moment.

Just as I turned back toward our room I saw a couple, walking briskly, bags all packed—with no baby. My heart sank. The possibilities ran through my head: "What could have happened to this couple?" I looked at my daughter and began to tear up. I knew something terrible had just happened. I prayed for this couple.

Thirteen days later I came across this story, your story, on the news. I'm quite certain that couple I saw was you. I read your story and was unusually moved to tears. Your openness, vulnerability, and awareness of strength found in the midst of

weakness—all this has strengthened me. That you find hope in
God's unshakable plan for you is a great encouragement to me.

I wonder why God crossed our paths if even for the briefest
of moments. You in your deepest pain, and me in great joy—all
by the nurses' desk. To be honest, I feel a very real, disconcerting
unfairness in this all. And although I want to, there is no way
for me to sense, even in the slightest, the dark corners of your
grief. So, hold fast to the hope of His promise. Hold fast.

I can't believe it. I cannot believe that this man knew us,
because my broken heart knew him. This man I have focused
my anger on is someone who wishes he could share our pain.
He is a father just like Aaron. His child, a child like Reid. And
after reading his words, I feel my unwavering rage start to lift.
I realize that I will never truly wish that he could know our
grief. He can't know it, but he certainly changed it. I want
to believe that if God did have a role in this encounter, and
crossed our paths, that it could be for this very reason.

● ☾ ●

IT IS TYPED out along the bottom:
Keepsake heart urn, tree of life $189
That's what the invoice reads. It was the original one we'd
chosen—the size they recommended for newborn babies. A
pale-green heart with a golden tree engraved into the stone.
I didn't love it, but it was better than the alternative, a minia-
ture urn with cherubs smiling down over it. That was before
we got the call.

"I'm so terribly sorry to say this." The man pauses to clear his throat. "But there's more of your son than we expected and he doesn't fit in the urn you chose. You'll need to come in and choose a new one."

It takes a minute to repeat his words in my mind before I can formulate some kind of answer. "There's more of him than you expected? How does that happen?" I put the call on speaker and place it on the coffee table for Aaron to hear.

"I'm so sorry. It all depends on the skeleton," he starts to explain. "You see, the bone density…" He clears his throat again. "It's a guessing game, really. Usually the keepsake urns are the perfect size. We could fill the urn and put the remainder in an envelope for you? If you're planning to get jewelry made, that might be a good option?"

"Could you please hold?" I press mute. I want to smash my phone into pieces. But I don't want Reid away from us for another day. I unmute the call, looking to Aaron to say something. "Could we come in again to speak to someone?" Aaron asks.

"Yes, of course. Anytime. No appointment needed."

We go to the funeral home the next day. The surprised look of an unfamiliar receptionist should have been our first clue. There isn't anyone there to help us. They bring out an assistant, and she shows us back to the room full of glass display cases featuring the various urns then waits nervously by the door. We stand by the wall with the keepsake urns for the babies and stare. I start to cry. Aaron suggests we just buy one, any one, and search for a better one on our own later.

Then the assistant speaks. "You know, I think I remember seeing some in the back. They're not the usual choice, but maybe..." She smiles shyly before hurrying out of the room.

She knocks softly on the door before returning. In her hands is a small wooden cylinder. It is clearly handmade, and on the top there is a spot carved out for a tea light. "They're made by a local company out of reclaimed wood," she starts to explain.

For Aaron, a man with woodworking in his blood, and me, a woman with an affinity for candles, it really does seem like an ideal fit. Reid, such a combination of both of us, would be at home in a beautiful combination of two things we love.

I don't need to look at Aaron to know he is smiling too. "It's great," he says. "That's the one."

6

WHEN MY BLEEDING tapers to a flow that no longer requires adult diapers and the hospital pill bottle containing my pain medication is empty, we decide it is time to leave the apartment, go somewhere other than the funeral home. For days I have been watching tiny bodies walk by from our window. Young men running fast, old men walking dogs, and occasionally, moms pushing strollers containing babies. I marvel at their ability to float through their everyday lives. When tragedy hits, everything pauses, and it's discomfiting to see that the whole world doesn't pause in solidarity. I watch anyway, as if within them there is some hidden secret, one that can help me return to a life where my son is alive. Then there is the weather: seemingly mocking when it's sunny, yet punishing when it rains. Though I do find some solace in the rain, as it more accurately reflects my mood.

We attempt our first walk around the block. We open the door to where our hall meets the elevator. It's empty, and that is comforting in a way I didn't know a bare space could be. The elevator takes us down and opens to sun blazing through the glass entrance doors. I have to squint to adjust to the light.

I wish I could say that the rays of sunshine lift my spirits, but it feels as if they are thrashing down against my back. I feel numb, apart from being aware of both the pain when I walk and Aaron's hand at the small of my back. We are both dressed in black, and our red-rimmed eyes stay hidden behind dark lenses. I feel like a shell of myself—my belly still soft and round, its emptiness shattering me. Still, I know I need to re-enter the world, even if only for a moment.

In the literature of grief, people talk about "second firsts"— the things you do for the first time after your loss, every action experienced anew in the light of what has happened. I wince with each step carrying me over every one of these second firsts, grasping that each one is taking me further away from the last time I held Reid. I wonder if the people passing us on the street notice the liquid streaming silently down my face.

As we wait for the light to change at the first crosswalk, a woman beams at us from her car. Her eagerness strikes me as nearly comical. She frantically rolls down her window, bobbing up and down with the manual stroke of each turn. Leaning ever so slightly out of her car, she suddenly yells at us: "My goodness! You two are beautiful!" She removes her own sunglasses and they dance around as she waves her hands animatedly through the air. "You're glowing! *Glowing*! There's just this amazing bright light surrounding you!" She sits there grinning and gaping at us.

I manage to return a half smile as I repeatedly press the button to cross, and Aaron gives her a soft wave. We then walk across the street as quickly as we can. I can't escape the situation fast enough, and yet I can't help but turn back. I watch that odd woman peer at us with her bright, happy eyes until the light turns green and she drives away. I keep watching, observing her blond hair whip around each time she turns her head to look back at us, until finally her car is just a speck in the distance on Granville Street.

After, I will wish I could ask that woman what she saw. I wonder if in some way she sensed Reid's spirit was near us. I can't pretend to know what happens after we die, but it doesn't seem so farfetched to me to think that our soul might linger. Is there a life between lives? If so, I find myself deliberating how long Reid might have stayed with us—whether out of a desire to protect or comfort or heal, or some other reason entirely, I don't know. No one does, do they? Are there any cold hard facts about life after death? It all comes down to faith, really. Belief—in something or nothing—is a choice. I decide I will choose to remain open, to not discount anything as coincidence, to hold space in my heart for all of the new and unforeseen ways our son might still be a part of our story.

● ☾ ●

APRIL LEAVES IN a blur. With it, we leave Reid's birth month behind and enter the next phase of anniversaries we don't want, milestones that should have been, and firsts we didn't anticipate. May 3, a month since his passing; May 4, which should have been his one-month birthday. I will the minutes and hours to slow down, but they refuse. I feel I have nothing to show for the time that has passed already.

That is the cruelest part, really. We spent nine months preparing for the biggest change of all—caring for a newborn. Right now, our world should be turned upside down by our efforts to learn how to burp after feeds and trim tiny nails and get milk stains out of shirts. But life carries on for us just as it did before Reid died. Although we know that everything is different in our hearts, at the same time everything is familiar in our routines. Everything has changed, yet nothing has changed. The new normal, with a sickening twist.

Aaron is back at work. He tells me that this is what he needs, asks if it's okay that he invites my mom to stop by during the days.

He sends me texts:

What are you doing?

How is your morning?

Are you eating?

I reply:

Oh, I'm very busy. What are YOU doing?

It's going. How's YOURS?

A little. Are YOU eating?

I keep waiting for the first day without tears to pass, but that day is still a long way off. Physically, I feel a bit like myself again, which is both comforting and terrifying: as my body begins to look and feel more like it did before pregnancy, I sense that I am leaving parts of Reid behind. Emotionally, though, I feel like a stranger in my own skin. The clarity I felt in the days after Reid's celebration has dissipated. As everyone starts to get back to their routines, as Aaron slowly returns to his, I am left without one, alone. And I feel lost.

My mom went on temporary leave from her job as a physio-therapist after Reid died. So now we spend the days walking around our neighborhood, searching for a new rental home when at first I can't stand to stay where we are. Then, when my feelings shift and I realize I can't leave the only place that knew him, we fill our time with matinées and spin classes. She sits on the couch with me in the mornings and listens as I spout off ideas for what I will do with my life now. She encourages me to apply for the yoga teacher training pro-gram I found last night, one that is scheduled to start in two months. She is, I think, the only reason I leave my bed at all.

Reid was my plan, the only one I ever really wanted to follow through on. For as long as I can remember I've had trouble determining what it is I want to do. Environmental science, modeling, art, biology, writing—all of these things I started but never fully committed to. I always felt drawn in another direction as soon as I'd settled on a particular path. I had decided to pull back from fashion, wanting to finish my science degree. But when I got pregnant, the formaldehyde exposure in my labs was a problem and I had to withdraw. It was fine, because the pregnancy, the child, it all felt right. *This* was what I was supposed to do; I was sure of it. Motherhood. I was so confident that it was what everything up until then was leading me toward.

Aaron and I weren't exactly well off, but I had earned a good living as a model, and we had some decent savings. Aaron had immersed himself in the local tech scene as a soft-ware developer, product manager, and coder, and was doing well. And once I was able to, I'd return to part-time model-ing. Otherwise I would stay home with Reid until he started school, and then I would go back myself, finish that degree. In the meantime, he would be my life. My happy, wanted, full life. So where was I going to find meaning now?

In the first weeks after Reid's death, I have long conversations with my dad about faith. Organized religion had never been a big part of my childhood, apart from three week-long summer Bible camps and Easters and Christmases at the Anglican church where I'd been baptized. My sisters and I would sit in a pew at the front with my maternal grandparents, wearing bows in our hair and matching outfits. After, at home, we would put said bows in our grandfather's hair, giggling at his feigned looks of terror.

My father never attended. It just became the norm, and after our questions about why were answered with, "He just doesn't come," we stopped asking.

I eventually found out the truth. My father had grown up in a strict Protestant community in a small town in the interior of British Columbia. When he was fifteen, he hitched a ride home with a stranger. That stranger took a sharp turn and flipped the truck in an accident that shattered my father's spine. All of the dreams he held for his future shattered with it. He was an all-star athlete and the whole town believed he was destined for great things in his sport. So they told him to pray. They urged him, "Pray hard, Ricky, and you'll walk again."

He did pray, but he never did walk. And there were members of his community who said it was because he didn't pray hard enough.

His faith changed after that accident, but he still believed in God. What changed was that he realized that your church—your place of worship—is in your heart. When he realized that—when he was able to see love, light, and hope in living with his challenge—he was able to see his community in this way too, forgiving them for blaming him.

When I talk to my dad after Reid's death, he tells me that he had a choice. He could have struggled to stay in the life he'd planned, but that no longer existed. Or he could choose to feel the pain, cling to hope, and lean on the support of others while searching for new goals and new dreams. The choice he made led to accomplishments beyond what anyone could have imagined. He won marathons, medaled at the Paralympics, and wheeled around the world. He dedicated himself to raising awareness and funds for those living with spinal cord injuries, to help with research and improving their quality of life.

Ask him today what he would have done if he had been given the option not to get in that pickup truck, knowing what he knows now, and he won't hesitate to tell you that he still would have taken that ride. He sees the accident, and the resulting disability (or as he would put it, *ability*), as one of his greatest blessings. His life was great before his accident, and it became even more incredible after. Not because of it—he didn't need to break his back to find his calling. But because he believed that his dreams were possible. What he accomplished was in him, through faith. But it was a faith that he found on his own terms, a faith free of judgment and an ask-and-receive God. A faith in a God devoted to nurturing us to thrive, not helping us decide who gets to. A faith in the good.

He tells me that all these years later, he knows that he would not be the same person—would not have grown, lived, and loved as much—if he hadn't gone through that terrible moment on June 27, 1973. He wouldn't have gone on his Man in Motion World Tour where he wheeled around the world and changed the lives of millions. He wouldn't have met my mother, or had me and my sisters, and Reid wouldn't have been born. He says that although it is hard for me to realize right now, and although Reid's life over those brief months was an absolute gift, his passing—in the most profound sense—might lead to the greatest miracle of all.

● ☾ ●

"HOW DID HE DIE?" the elderly woman in line behind me asks. Small talk about her pregnant daughter around my age led to a conversation about babies, which led to the question about whether I have children. I said that I have a son, but he died.

"He was stillborn at forty weeks," I reply. "A knot in his umbilical cord."

"Oh!" She gives me a tight smile and then says, "You know, I forgot to grab something. Excuse me."

She turns around and leaves, and I am left standing with my cart full of groceries, trying to process what just happened. She sounded *relieved*. As if stillbirth wasn't so bad.

I'm learning that people find it difficult to talk about dead babies. But I don't want it to be difficult to talk about Reid. I don't want him to be a secret to hide away, or an uncomfortable truth to keep to myself. I want to do something that publicly recognizes the place he holds in our lives. I just don't know what.

Aaron and I are away for the weekend, visiting a mountainside town just outside the city. We decide to go on a bike ride, which for my still-bleeding postpartum body isn't proving to be the most comfortable activity. After a few too many bumps in the unpaved road, we pull our bikes off the path and find a spot by the lake to sit and talk. The one-month mark is fast approaching, and we don't know what to do.

"I want to do something to remember him," I say, picking at a piece of grass stuck in my laces. "Remember the time we had with him. And I don't know that saying 'he should have been one month old' feels right."

"I get that," he says. "But it's also true."

"Well, I hate that it's true." And I do. I love him, and I can't bear that I have to prove that love because the only time we got with him was during my pregnancy. I need that time to hold weight. I need it to count.

"Remember those tie stickers?" Aaron asks. We were going to take pictures of him every month with the numbered tie-shaped stickers, so that we could document how much he grew.

"I'd forgotten about those!" An idea is starting to form in my head. "What about doing something to honor the months of my pregnancy with him?" I grab my phone and he scoots closer to me, glancing at my screen.

We brainstorm ideas; look through my calendar, old photos, text messages. Eventually, we end up with a list of places we were and people we were with on the fourth day of each month of my pregnancy. We are amazed to realize that each date involves a member of our community, and that everyone is included by month nine.

"What if we recreate parts of these days," Aaron suggests, "and—"

"Leave the stickers there?" I interrupt, knowing exactly what he's thinking.

That's it. That's what we need. We come up with a hashtag for the project: #ninemonthswithreid. And we don't care that this is focused on the past. That's where our son lives, and nine months seems like a short amount of time to meet with him there again.

When I had been pregnant with Reid for one month, we walked to Granville Island with some of our dearest friends. We hadn't told them I was pregnant yet, but I was giving it away with my intense craving for an icy vanilla-flavored drink. I wanted to stop for one on our way down, but nobody wanted to chance missing the sunset. When we got to the water, we sat on the benches and watched the sky subdue to milky hues of orange and pink as we talked. It felt significant, and I was glad we hadn't missed it.

When we finally left and went to get my drink we learned that the store had closed early that day. I cried on the sidewalk in front of the store, sulked the whole way back to our apartment. Our friends averted their eyes, pretended the scene I'd just caused didn't happen. Later I could laugh about it, and poke fun at them for not realizing that I was pregnant.

On May 4 this year, we go back to Granville Island with the same friends, except this time I get my drink first. I sit on the same bench where we watched the sunset all those months ago, remembering what it was like to carry a soul within my own. Aaron turns to me and suggests that this bench is the place we should leave his sticker, on the beam between us.

As we remove the glossy backing from the one-month tie, Aaron wipes away the tears from behind his sunglasses, and the sight of him forces me to do the same. We lay the sticker against the cool metal post. I kiss the tips of my fingers and press them to the center of it, smoothing out the wrinkles. We smile. And then we laugh, out loud, for the first time since his death. I feel mortified, like we are undermining the magnitude of our loss. But our grief is on its own timeline, and laughter is just what we need today.

The next week, Rebecca takes the day off to spend it with me—"We can do whatever you want," she says—and we walk along the beach toward Granville Island, taking the path to the wharf where I put Reid's first sticker. When we arrive at the bench, the sticker is still there.

"I wasn't expecting that," Rebecca marvels. "It's amazing. That it survived the hail storm and all the rain." Then she points to a toddler down the dock peeling happy-face stickers from another bench. "And that it survived *that.*" We laugh, and then I start to cry and she wraps me up in her arms.

Of all my family and friends, Rebecca was the most outwardly excited for Reid to be born. As a preschool teacher, she lives and breathes children. Throughout my pregnancy, she lobbied for babysitting rights and bought assortments of tiny outfits and toys. I relished her joy, and the experience that had finally managed to close the gap of our age difference.

Rebecca and I will often walk this route together over the next months, and the sticker will always be there. Years later, it will be gone, but its persistence feels meaningful to me.

● ☾ ●

PREGNANT BELLIES ARE all around me. At the bakeshop I
frequent, crossing the sidewalk, appearing in the bookstore
aisle. I want to run from them. I want to look down and see
the same roundness. Mostly, I want to cry out warnings.

One thought plays over and over on a loop in my mind:
I should have protected him. That was my job—to grow, nurture, and defend him. I had a responsibility to protect him.
But what should have been the safest place for Reid was in fact
full of unsuspected danger. My body failed.

I think back constantly to the day before his death—that
last full, simple, naively joyful day of my life. I slept in that
morning because Reid had kept me up with his gymnastics,
and only rolled out of bed when it was time to get ready for
prenatal yoga. The sun was shining, the blossoms were out in
full force, and life was a sweet waiting game. It was a day like
any other. No signs of impending tragedy. Just a collection
of average moments made extraordinary by the life I carried
inside me.

After yoga that morning I went to the grocery store to
shop for dinner. I was texting Aaron to get his opinion and
sending photos from the aisles as I browsed. The last photo
in my camera roll before Reid's passing and birth is a photo
of the food we ended up eating that night. It seems so silly. I
wish it were something epic, like a bump photo or a portrait
from our slow and happy days. But it's just a photo from my
trip to the market. I contemplate deleting photos so the last
one will be something more important, but I am coming to
cherish this reminder that all was normal then; all was well.

That evening we had our friend Jonny over for dinner, and after the meal, we put *Interstellar* on. At around midnight, I got three very intense kicks from Reid—the most willful I'd ever felt him give. In that moment, I remember thinking to myself: *He's getting so strong!* I turned to Jonny and asked if he wanted to feel. He shyly opted not to, and I chuckled at his reaction and told him, "It's fine, you'll have plenty of time to play once he's out." Eventually, I caved to exhaustion, but just before I got up, Jonny put his hand on my belly and said, "Goodnight, Reid."

I don't think I felt him move again after that.

With the gifts that the perspective of passing time gives, hard truths come too. My mind is starting to recall new things as the shock that protected me initially wears thin. Now I wonder if one of his wiggles that day was him accidentally pulling the knot tight. If those three kicks were his last struggles for oxygen. If that was him suffocating.

I don't believe there is one specific moment I can pinpoint to say, "Aha! There! That's where we swoop in and save our son." Though there are times I think, "Well, maybe there?" Had I known that those three urgent kicks could have been out of panic, that this tiny deviation from his normal movements could have been a warning, would it have changed anything? Will I always wonder if one thing or another could have altered his fate? Was there some point where I could have made a trade: my life for his? I have to believe in my heart that nothing could have saved his life, because I can't change anything now. But my mind will always question it. Because I am his mother and I should have known. *I should have known.*

What I am feeling, I realize, looks a lot like survivor's guilt. When I look at our photos from the later weeks of pregnancy, I can't help but feel that we look so silly, smiling and laughing with naive joy. It should have been us who died—us with decades of life behind us. How could we not see that death was just around the corner? I try to warn that oblivious couple: "Get him out! Get him out *now!*" But of course, the people in the photos can't hear me through the glossy barrier of time.

I have to practice forgiveness, I know. I have to make peace with my body. After all, she did everything she was designed to do. That knot was no one's fault; it was an accident, a terrible accident. So for Reid, and for myself, I make a silent vow to stop drowning in guilt and shouting at photos. The past can't save me. It will never look any different.

I wander over to my mat, something I've been doing a lot lately. Yoga allows me to feel close to Reid. When I go through the same poses and motions that I did in prenatal class, repeat the same mantras, it's not so difficult to remember what life was like before death. I keep coming back to the same mantra, one that the instructor used often: *Sa Ta Na Ma*. I try to remember exactly what she said it meant. Something about birth, life, death, and rebirth. The sounds are nice to say, and regardless of the meaning they feel appropriate. As I whisper them over and over, making circles with my torso while on my hands and knees, they bring comfort. I am here moving, living, making progress. And one day, I can do these things away from the safety of this rubber rectangle.

● ☾ ●

MOTHER'S DAY IS tomorrow, May 10. My first Mother's Day—now one without my child to hold. I *am* a mother, but what kind of mother am I? My claim seems less certain after death. I read a quote by Donald Winnicott, a British pediatrician and psychoanalyst, saying, "There is no such thing as a baby. There exists a mother-infant pair." He was talking about this in terms of psychotherapy, looking at people relationally and at the significance of the bond between a mother and her child, but this description extended to the connection established during pregnancy. I also read about the British psychologist John Bowlby and his studies on the early mother-child relationship, which concluded "not only that attachment behaviour is necessary for survival but also that it is core, intrinsic, and genetically built in."[2] This bond is so strong that in psychotherapy it is considered different from any other.

If this mother-child relationship, this identity, is ingrained in us at a genetic level, I just can't believe that death would simply sever it. Death wouldn't change anything at all. Except that one of us is here and the other there, and though the circumstances are altered, the connection will never be. The mother will always remain a mother; the child, her child.

Still, I know the day will be difficult on my grieving heart. Aaron and I leave town and go off the grid, not sure how to face other families out celebrating.

In the morning, he makes me pancakes and I try to honor the day. I trace the line of my linea nigra, still dark on my belly, evidence of the mother-infant pair that Reid and I are. I leave room for sorrow too, knowing that it will come to the party whether invited or not.

● ☾ ●

TWO YEARS INTO our relationship, and a year after finishing high school, I enrolled at the Christian university Aaron was attending to start my science degree. I'd taken a gap year after graduation to model full time, spending most of it abroad. I missed Aaron and wanted to be close to him again—long-distance was taking a toll on us, our communications restricted to emails and calling in the small windows when our respective time zones lined up. I also wanted to learn more about this faith he'd been raised in, explore ways I might be able to integrate my own faith in science with one in religion.

At the end of the year, on a stormy Good Friday at the start of final exams, Aaron and I took a break from studying and walked down to the quaint riverside town near the school. We strolled along the river, lukewarm coffees from the resident bookstore café in hand. It had just started to pour when we reached the end of the boardwalk that looked out over the water; mist fanned over it in every direction.

"What's on your mind?" Aaron asked. He could tell I was somewhere else with my thoughts.

"The more I learn at this school," I started, "the more I feel that there is something bigger than me."

He looked at me inquisitively. I sat down on the wet planks of the boardwalk, the rain soaking through my layers, and motioned for him to sit next to me. "I've been thinking about it a lot," I continued. "I believe in God. I want what I do with my life to be in service of others."

"I'm sensing a but?" he said.

I smiled. "But—" I tried to find my wording. "But I don't know enough about Christianity to have faith in it all. Don't people spend their entire lives leaning into the scriptures and turning them over and analyzing their validity?"

"That's true," he replied. "I don't think the point is that you have it all figured out before you commit to faith. That's a little counterintuitive to what faith is."

I laughed. I hadn't actually realized that I had been trying to prove the faith first, before I could say I believed.

Then he told me, "I think the idea is that there are things that we don't know, and that you learn more as you pursue God in your life."

So I decided, right then and there, wet from the rain and the beginnings of tears, to make that promise. I said aloud the words belonging to the prayer that would signify my commitment to a lifelong relationship with God. The feeling overcame me, and the choice came after.

I still didn't agree with the entirety of the Bible, or at least not with people's interpretations of it. But I believed in God, and wanted to pursue that relationship, work to understand His teachings, aspire to live a life rooted in love. Because there was so much more to gain for others and myself than if I went with the alternative—lived as if God and His word weren't real, and discovered after death that I was wrong.

Exactly five years after that Good Friday when I became a Christian, my son died. Then Saturday came and he was born still. We first believed a miracle was possible, given the connection. But there was no miracle for us, or at least not the one we expected. I think about how the friends and loved ones of Jesus grieved His passing on a Saturday too, not knowing that Sunday would come bringing celebration. I often wonder why our Easter Sunday never came.

I wonder if instead I received a punishment—retribution for not declaring complete and total trust in the Bible five years ago. Somewhere along the way I'd stopped actively seeking God. I'd reached a place where it didn't seem as urgent. Life was good. We were comfortable and content to stay that way. Maybe that was the problem.

7

T IS JUNE, and I am on a plane to Winnipeg, Manitoba. I am here on a leap of faith, really. Many readers who wrote to me after my post about Reid's death suggested that I meet a woman named Amelia Barnes. Amelia is a shop owner and yoga instructor who lost her firstborn son, Landon, last summer, three days after he was born. I was hesitant but sent her a message introducing myself and sharing my story.

Now I am traveling to a remote lake in a faraway province, headed to Landon's Legacy Healing Retreat along with dozens of other women who have lost children too. I have no idea what to expect. I have connected with so many strangers online, but never face-to-face. I never thought I'd travel halfway across the country for something I found out about on Instagram. But so many "never thoughts" have already come to pass, so why not one more?

I am moving forward now, deliberately. Sitting here in row 14 by myself, I see the moment clearly. This trip is a testament to the work I am willing to do to experience healing in this post-loss world, because it is so out of character. At least, for the old me. Perhaps the new me does things of this sort all the time.

I think back to an interview I did years ago, when I was applying for admission to a fine arts university. I had wanted to study painting, but one of the interviewers called me "suburban and safe." They didn't mean those things as compliments. Their words stuck with me even after I was accepted, and I turned down the offer. Technically, they were talking about my art, but there really isn't much difference between art and self; in fact, art might be the truest expression of self. If I were to paint my soul now, it wouldn't be suburban. It certainly wouldn't be safe.

Amelia's mother meets me and four other moms attending the retreat at the airport and drives us out to the lake where the accommodations are. There is no small talk; immediately, we share our stories. When it is my turn I break down before any words can escape me. Another mom fetches Kleenex from her bag. "I never go anywhere without it anymore," she says.

I take a minute, and then I talk about Reid, stopping to soak up the tears with the tissue. I tell them about the knot in his cord and the pain in saying goodbye and the utter confusion about my place in the world that I feel now.

"When was he born?" asks another mom who also lost her daughter to a cord accident before birth.

"Ten weeks ago," I reply. "April fourth." There is a collective gasp from the women in the car. Doubt ripples through me. Am I doing this too soon?

I meet Amelia soon after we arrive at the lodge. We walk down to the water together, and the moment I look into her eyes I know: she understands my pain. There is tremendous power in that. Nothing needs to be said out loud. I just know.

Amelia is pregnant again. She tells the group before the retreat, acknowledging that this might be a trigger for some. I find myself drawn to her swelling belly, out of both fear and love. It seems incredible that she is functioning, not to mention leading a retreat for those who have lost babies. I am sure that when—or *if*—I become pregnant again, I will admit myself to the hospital to be monitored until the baby is born. Over the next few days, I will have to stop myself from shouting at her: "Watch out!" as she walks down a wet riverbank, or "Be careful!" as she flows swiftly in yoga, or "Should you eat that?" as she reaches for Caesar salad. Because what do I know about keeping babies safe? So I say nothing and just observe.

Later that night, we all gather for the first time. We form a circle in the loft above the dining hall. We've been asked to bring photos to place on an altar, but I'm not ready to print any of Reid yet—his image feels too raw and too sacred to me. The pictures are placed in the middle of our circle and we are asked to walk around and look at each one.

I feel sick. I don't see them as children, and that makes me feel guilty. I see twenty bodies who now don't have spirits. Before Reid died I'd never seen a corpse; now I've seen hundreds, from the parents who read my blog and send them my way. Not all of them were stillborn, but I can't manage to separate the image of them from the image I have of my own dead son.

Before we gathered, I had been lying in the bed in my room, looking up flights back home. I'm not sure I should be here. I think it's a mistake that I've come. It's all too big and too scary. It makes this *real*.

Then, as we circle around the photos of our children, the heavens open up outside and it pours. Tears roll down our cheeks and the rain comes down harder still. The sounds of our voices rise to be heard over the thunder and lightning strikes through the looming darkness. As we sit, after the last person has introduced herself and her child, and we have finally finished sharing, we look to the sky through the windows. A beautiful sunset with pink and purple hues peeks through the heavy clouds. Then, a golden butterfly soars across the window above Amelia's head. We all sit in awe. I'll give it one more day.

The next day before yoga, we practice compassionate listening. We are put in pairs and take turns sharing something we explored in our journaling. When it is our turn to listen, we are told to look into our partner's eyes for a minute without saying or doing anything. No comforting or physical touch is allowed. Eye contact is terrifying to me. But as someone who is more of a writer than a talker, I discover there is something wonderful about sitting in silence with someone as they share their most intimate thoughts. No drawing on your own experiences to try to relate, no giving advice, no trying to make it better. Just giving space for them to feel.

A guest speaker earlier this morning told us, "To fully heal from suffering you need to fully feel." Then, after stopping to gaze at each of us: "But grief isn't something you get through or get over." She paused for effect. "You live into it." It will take me years to understand what those words mean, but they will become words to live by.

Later that day, on a whim, we go to the Bannock Point Petroforms. The groundskeeper, who is serendipitously there, takes us to one of the large rock formations he particularly likes. He says it had been causing him trouble lately. He would arrange it in one shape—a turtle or a mountain—and by the following morning it would be changed to the shape of a pregnant woman. This had been going on for weeks and he couldn't figure out who or what was changing it. Finally, he decided to leave it. He tells us that when he looked more closely, he realized that it was a pregnant woman who had lost a child. We are all silent. He doesn't know our stories.

On our way back, he is sharing advice he has learned over the years. I am half listening, half looking out for ticks (Lyme disease is rare, but what does *rare* really mean to me anymore?) when I hear him say, "You know, the only thing you truly own are your words; when you give them, you bring honor." His words strike me; in our meditation workshop yesterday, when we were asked why we were here, I said that I wanted to gain the strength to find a way to honor Reid. I wonder if words might be a way I can do both.

The days start to blend together. We do workshops with healers and craniosacral therapy and counseling. We take an Ayurvedic lesson. I do my first postpartum handstand.

Being both the youngest mom and the one with the most recent loss is challenging, but in many ways it is also a tremendous blessing. My grief is so new, but to talk about Reid and my experience so openly, in a way I can't do anywhere else, feels transformative. The other women tell me I am brave to be here so soon. I don't see it that way. To me, they are the brave ones. Each woman here has been through hell and is fighting her way back to life. Each one of them inspires me. Through them I witness what my path might look like weeks, months, and years ahead, and it gives me the confidence to continue on.

Before I know it, it is time for the closing ceremony. We chant a mantra and build a mandala by the water. We move the altar of photos next to it, and among them I place the silver bean necklace I bought when I found out I was pregnant with Reid.

Later that afternoon, I post the lyrics to a song by Conn Bernard titled "Look for Me in Rainbows" to Instagram alongside a photo of me sitting on the lakeside dock looking out at a sunset. Minutes later, a beautiful rainbow appears in the sky. The other women and I all stand there marveling, knowing what I just shared online. It is another moment out of many where nature seems to be moving with us as we work through our grief. It isn't really a question of believing in signs. They are all around.

After, we build a bonfire behind the lodge and sit near its blaze. Some of the women sip wine, while some of us, myself included, choose tea from the convenience store. Alcohol makes us decidedly too emotional since our losses, we agree.

Amelia and I stand off to the side and look at the group in front of us. I ask her how it was for her, leading the retreat.

She starts to say all of the expected things, that it has been emotional and rewarding and powerful, and then stops. "It's actually been really hard as well. I feel like I've stepped into the role of leader and haven't had the chance to be a mother who has lost her child too."

I nod, though I don't really understand. "Are you nervous about being pregnant again?" I have wanted to ask her for days.

She rubs her belly and smiles, and after a deep inhale she says, "You know, I'm not. I want this baby to have the same experience as Landon. I did everything I could to keep him safe and feeling loved, and I know I'll do the same with his little sibling."

We continue to talk well after everyone else has gone to bed. We share some hard truths, things we've both been wrestling with: how much we want our children here with us, yet how different and somehow compelling our new paths are. We are no longer comfortable with "comfortable," and what we crave from life has expanded. The process of mourning the death of our firstborns is allowing us to gain a deeper sense of who we truly are, and we see how our hearts beat for more than ourselves. But then, are we just thinking this to try to find relief from the excruciating pain? Is that relief even possible?

We talk about what our children have given us: lessons in compassion and gifts of patience. When we finally get to parent an earth-side child, we imagine, we'll be completely different than we might have been with our sons. A full night of diaper changes, feeds, and crying sounds like the best thing in the world to us. We'd give anything to be experiencing the sleep exhaustion others talked about. The spit-up milk? We want that too. We aren't sure we would have felt the same had things gone another way. That isn't to say we think parents who haven't lost children aren't grateful in those moments too, but we can't speak to that. Loss is all we know.

I think about this for some time as I stand beside her in front of the flames, silent. Though I don't particularly like what we are confessing to each other, I know that on some level we are right. A part of me is sure that while I would have loved Reid endlessly, I would have been a different parent to him than the one I am imagining myself to be after his loss. Because I'm not sure I'd have instinctively left my selfish world, full of entitlement and privilege, where everything revolved around me. I didn't know that losing him was possible back then, but now that I do, I can't deny that it shifted my entire perspective on what was difficult but still so good, and what was just plain hard.

At the end of the retreat we say our tearful goodbyes, though this isn't really farewell. We know the relationships we have formed will last a lifetime, but also, our experiences have given us a different outlook on physical parting. We know that time doesn't create the bonds we form in this life. That memories of a single moment can last forever. That goodbye isn't the right word.

On the plane ride home, the woman next to me makes small talk. I've had very little patience for it lately, and when she asks if I had a nice time in Winnipeg, I am ready to dismiss her, say it was okay. But I want to test out my newfound confidence in talking about Reid, so I tell her why I was there.

"Oh honey, I'm so sorry," she says. Then she looks me in the eyes and asks, "Are you a believer?"

I'm not sure what she is asking if I believe in, but assuming she means God, I nod and say that I am. She lets out a relieved little exhale as she places her hand on my shoulder and assures me, "Then you'll see him again." She smiles and turns back to her book. It is as simple as that.

● ☾ ●

TODAY IS FATHER'S DAY. It's been two days since I've been home from Winnipeg, and I haven't given myself much time to consider Aaron's grief. I'm too preoccupied with my own. When I first got home, I asked Aaron how it was to go to church without me.

"Barb asked how you were doing," he said.

"That's sweet of her," I replied. "What did you say?"

"I told her you were at a healing retreat. That you were doing okay. She said that sounded like a nice opportunity."

"How did you say you were doing?" My indirect way of asking him myself.

"I didn't," he answered.

"What do you mean?"

He shrugged. "She didn't ask."

I hadn't realized how his grief was mostly going unrecognized. Because I had physical ties to Reid, maybe it appeared that I was the only one who was grieving, and somehow, the fact that we had both lost a child was overlooked. But he helped create and grow and birth our son too, and though Reid isn't in his arms right now he is still a father. I see it even more clearly now, and I hope I knew it during those forty weeks. He was a father when his warm arms wrapped around my hips as he brought his hands to my belly. He was a father when his fingers danced with Reid's little feet that kicked at his presence. He was a father when he cupped his hands around my belly button to talk to our son in that deep voice of his.

He was a father when he pleaded with Reid in that hospital room to kick one more time, just for him. He was a father when, through agonizing contractions, he told me, "You can do this," knowing each one brought us closer to seeing our child. He was a father when he cut the umbilical cord as Reid lay upon my chest.

He was a father when he talked to the funeral home director and made all of the arrangements. He was a father when he picked the beautiful handmade wooden urn. He was a father when he carefully put Reid's things back in his nursery and quietly shut the door.

He was a father then and he is still a father. His claim to that title is as valid as mine is to motherhood. It is only the way we express our parenthood that is different.

I am glad to be home but at the same time I want to be back at the retreat. I want to immerse myself again in a room full of people who know what it is I'm feeling without having to name it or pick it apart. I want to listen to their wise tales of experience from a life lived after loss.

For the most part, Aaron seems fine, and this makes me angry, though I don't understand it. I don't want him to struggle, but I'm angry he's fine. There it is. The unsettled gut, something acidic like jealousy responsible. People ask how we are doing, and I say that we are on the same page in our grief. I say we are okay, that I'm grateful. For a while this is the truth, but something has shifted since I've come home. So now I am lying, though not entirely. When we have conversations about Reid we agree how shitty it is that he's dead and how we want him back and we don't know what any of this means. The difference is that Aaron finds the magical powers necessary to get up and dressed and go to work, while I am mostly baffled by the first task. I don't know if we are on the same page, but we aren't worse off than the day Reid died, so that must count for something.

I do know that there is no shouting, no substance abuse, no visible sign of crisis. He really does seem fine. He is coping. And here I am, pissed that he is fine and coping while I'm about two more sleepless nights away from alerting the press and walking into a hair salon and shaving my head. That's how I'm doing.

But I don't want to think about me, not right now. Today I decide that I will study Aaron. This helps; obsessing over something other than how I'm doing is a relief. I note that Aaron leaves for work around seven thirty in the morning. He returns at around six thirty. He works at a tech start-up so the hours are long, but I believe he stretches his hours longer. I am not so far gone as to be oblivious to the fact that I'm not presently the most excellent company. He wraps me in a hug when he returns. He cooks dinner (I don't know when I last touched the stove). He doesn't ask how my day was, and for that I actually am grateful. I ask how his was, though. I listen to him talk about the office politics, the friends he has there, the keg that was installed in the lunchroom. We eat the dinner he made and I'm sure it is delicious, he is an excellent cook, but everything tastes a little bit like sand. He asks if I want to watch an episode of something with him, and I do. After, we have sex on the couch. We go to bed, kiss goodnight, turn our backs to each other. He says he loves me. I say I love him too.

The whole day, he seems fine. But he must not be. There is no *fine* after your baby dies. He must feel that if he is anything other, we will not make it. Someone has to steer this ship, and it's not going to be me. I know it's not fair. But what is?

● ☾ ●

HEALING AFTER LOSING a child isn't a linear progression, though I initially believed otherwise. There aren't "steps" to grief, nor is there any "completion" of it. And the saying "time heals all wounds" doesn't apply when your baby dies. I doubt it applies to any loss. I doubt the healing is ever done.

Elisabeth Kübler-Ross, the famous psychiatrist who established the five stages of grief, was a name I had a vague awareness of. After Reid died, I searched out her work and tried to make my own grief follow these stages. For the first while, it seemed I was on track. When I was done with denial, I would move on to anger, then from anger to bargaining. When it was time for depression I was confused, because I had been in constant tears and was restless in my feelings of hopelessness right from the start. Suddenly I'd be back at denial, or somewhere else entirely. I was convinced there was something wrong with me. I kept trying to work to achieve acceptance, to say I'd arrived there, and then to one day actually believe it.

I later learned that Dr. Kübler-Ross's stages were never meant to be applied as a one-size-fits-all model. They were first observed under circumstances of anticipatory grief in cancer patients, and later in their loved ones, but were never intended to be used generally, and never intended to control the feelings of grief or prescribe the order these feelings should follow. But they became the cultural and professional belief and were strictly applied to the entire spectrum of loss.

The stages are being examined more closely now, though. Counselors and psychotherapists, most of whom have known loss intimately and found that their own experiences didn't connect to the rigid use of the five stages, are working to normalize grief, to reveal where we are falling short on our theories and the application of them.

Megan Devine, a grief counselor who lost her partner, and the author of *It's OK That You're Not OK*, discusses Kübler-Ross's stages in her book:

> *The stages of grief were not meant to tell anyone what to feel and when exactly they should feel it. They were not meant to dictate whether you are doing your grief "correctly" or not. Her stages, whether applied to the dying or those left living, were meant to normalize and validate what someone might experience in the swirl of insanity that is loss and death and grief. They were meant to give comfort, not create a cage...*
>
> *...You can't force an order on pain. You can't make grief tidy or predictable. Grief is as individual as love: every life, every path, is unique. There is no pattern, and no linear progression. Despite what many "experts" believe, there are no stages of grief. Despite what the wider population believes, there are no stages of grief.*

One afternoon, a few weeks after the retreat, I clean the apartment. I wash the sheets and scrub the bathroom and open up all the windows. I am feeling relatively good. Then, as I'm dusting, my brush glides across Reid's urn. I stop, frozen mid-action. I am dusting my son. *Dusting him.*

I burst into tears. I don't think I've ever really tried to grasp the reality that his remains are inside. I can't bring myself to process it. I am mostly okay when I think about him still being present in our lives in some way, when I can picture him somewhere like heaven, looking over his loved ones. But now that I understand, for the first time, that his physical body is in something I have to dust, I am weak from the pain of it, pierced through with anxiety. There are parts of me that don't yet understand that he is dead. I have to learn this again and again and again. At the glimpse of a photo or during a conversation with a stranger or when I dust his urn.

I shouldn't have to dust my child. It is all so awful and terrible, and I hate that this is my story. I hate that this is Reid's story. I don't care about the good shining through this darkness. It just really fucking sucks. There is no order to any of this, no predictability, no cure. I think that's the truth many fear the most.

● ☾ ●

I DECIDE TO return to work. Modeling is something I've always had an ebb-and-flow relationship with, but it is the one thing I can add to my days immediately. My agent, Liz Bell, supports my return, saying whatever size I am is fine (something I've always loved her for—advocating for inclusivity in an industry where a specific size is usually a requirement to work). So my mom and I go shopping—I need clothes that fit my postpartum curves. We drive into Gastown and, for fun, browse luxury pieces in classic white, black, and gray: my color palette. We look for a while, fingering the fabrics, and then make our way to the change rooms.

"Emma? Here's your room," says the saleswoman.

Another woman turns around and stares at me for a moment before asking, "Emma Hansen?"

I smile and say yes.

Sensing that I'm not connecting the dots, she explains that she used to work for a clothing label I'd shot for years ago. "Someone told me recently that you were about to have a baby! Oh, who was that..." She trails off as she puts her finger to her mouth. "Oh well. Anyway, congrats!" She beams.

Congrats. That's something I've had yet to hear when the conversation is about my son. Clearly, she hasn't heard the full story, but I don't care. It feels nice to be congratulated. This is what it must be like for parents who have living children.

I have to say something; we work in the same circles and she'll find out anyway, so I simply say, "Thank you, yes, I did. But he passed away in April."

Her eyes dart to the floor as tears start to fill them. "I'm so sorry," she says. She fiddles with the button on her sleeve and explains, "I have a son. I just..." She puts her hand on my forearm, something people tend to do a lot as of late. I don't know why, but I want to give her a big hug. I stop myself, because I barely know her and it feels like an inappropriate response, but she looks so devastated.

One of the gifts of Amelia's retreat is that now I'm able to talk freely about my son—his life and his death. I am oddly okay in this moment, out in public, having this conversation with a relative stranger. Following our birth story going viral, I haven't yet run into someone who didn't know what happened, so I stopped anticipating the possibility. I never thought I'd be congratulated on the birth of my son. The congrats never came, but I still had a son. My body conceived him, grew him, birthed him. I wish I heard it more often.

8

I T WAS THE second weekend in July, one year ago. Hanah, Micaela, and I were sipping gin and tonics with mint; the dock rocked us up and down as we lay in the sun.

I was daydreaming, thinking back to the night before with Aaron. We were still newlyweds then, having just returned home after our extended honeymoon of living and working in New York. His strong, tanned arms had quickly found their way around my waist and as he undressed me, he paused, pressing me gently against the wall. Our lips met earnestly. It was a moment we couldn't let slip away from us. It all came easily then. The passion, the love, the intimacy.

Hanah had just put the rendition of "No Angels" by Bastille on the speakers—it was on repeat that summer—and brought her drink up to her lips, pausing to touch her nose. It was the first thing to go numb when she drank, a quirk of hers. I watched her fondly from the edge of the dock.

We were drunk on more than just the wine; youth spilled out of us, seeping into the warmth of that Pacific summer air. When the sun went down, before the buzz of the day started to wear thin, we stripped away our clothes as we ran to meet the ocean. It was freezing. The other two left the water in a hurry, but I stayed. I let the seaweed travel the length of my limbs, feeling the numbing effects of the liquid both inside and outside of me. I looked up to the sky and was taken aback by the moon, by how striking it was. Its fullness from the night before was evident. And I couldn't put my finger on it, but something about that moment felt significant. Significant enough that I lingered in the cold, unable to take my eyes off the moon in the sky.

What I didn't know then was that just below my belly button, mere inches beneath the surface of my skin, a very real, very new life was forming. A child was conceived on that July full moon, much like the full blood moon he'd be born on months later. A cycle guided by moonlight, remembered by it, too.

With that memory, another set of anniversaries starts. July 12, the anniversary of Reid's conception. I wonder how long my years will revolve around these dates, in nine-month cycles. This first one sends me back into a depression. I miss him.

I decide that I need to get a tattoo of Reid's name; I need him to be a visible part of me somehow. Aaron wants to get one too. When we were living in New York, he got our wedding date tattooed on his leg. He had this idea that he would add the birthdays of our future children above it, creating a line up his calf. We used to joke that once the type got to knee level we'd have to stop having children because it would look weird to go any higher.

I call around to tattoo parlors and ask if they have any drop-in appointments available, but they keep saying they're booked. As I'm calling, I send pictures back and forth to family and friends. I'm fairly set on script style until I stumble across a delicate typewriter font. Yes, that's it. For all the words I've written for my son and all the words that have yet to come.

Finally, maybe sensing the desperation in my voice, some-one on the other end of the line asks, "What is this tattoo for?"

"I just want my son's name on my body. My husband wants his birth date," I answer. Then I add, "He died."

I think the line is disconnected; there is silence for a few moments. At last the person says, "I'm so sorry for your loss. Can you be here in thirty minutes?"

The artist's station is immaculate, completely sterile and free of clutter. He has photos of his work up on the wall behind his chair, and a few that look like family portraits. Aaron, sensing my nerves, offers to go first. As the artist preps Aaron's leg, shaves a small rectangle, I think to ask how many memorial tattoos he's done, but I don't have the courage. He starts up his tattoo gun and I study Aaron's face as the needle pierces his skin. It remains unchanged. Twenty minutes later, the tattoo is done. It matches his first exactly.

Then I am on the table holding my arm out for a complete stranger to permanently alter. I close my eyes. I'm surprised that I don't feel any pain. It isn't long before the artist says he is done and I peek down to examine the new addition to my body. I smile: the base of the r is slightly slanted. A little

imperfection that will serve as a simple reminder that I don't
have control. I never have and I never will. And now, I look
at my wrist and I think of my son. *Reid*. The one word that
says it all.

● ☾ ●

MY YOGA TEACHER training has started. At first, it's strange
to sit in a room with twenty-eight other people who know
nothing about me, Reid, or my story. In a way, it is nice to
not be defined by my loss. Sometimes I've wished I could
share the "Reid" part without the "Reid's bereaved mother"
part. As I've slowly started to enter back into my community, I've noticed that I am very much "the woman whose
baby died," and when you're that woman, people often cease
to include you in their conversations about pregnancy and
parenthood the way they would have had things turned out
differently.

One day, I am in a room with a group of extended family and friends, sipping on wine, when the mothers in the
group start sharing their birthing stories. The question "Did
you poop?" comes up. Everyone is in fits of laughter as each
woman shares her own experience, then turns to the next
woman and asks her to share hers.

No one asks me. There's an awkward silence when the
mother beside me is finished talking, and an abrupt change in
the conversation. I could interrupt, tell my story too, chuckle
and say, "They said I didn't but, *phew*, my body sure cleared
itself out when labor started." But I know they won't hear my
answer the way I ache for them to.

If I can't tell these stories, can't connect with other people as a parent, I'm not sure where I fit. Losing Reid didn't mean I stopped seeing myself as a mother, but if other people don't see me that way—if there is no public sign of my motherhood—can I really claim that identity? And if I'm not a mother, then who does that make Reid?

A woman in my training comes up to me at the end of class one day and says, "So you're a mother! How old is your kid?"

We were asked earlier to write down three titles we identified with, then introduce ourselves to each other using them. I wrote down:

I am a mother
I am a wife
I am a writer

I try to prepare the woman with a look before I reply, "He would have been three months."

She mishears me. "Three months? Wow!"

"No." I shake my head. "He *would* have been three months. He passed away in April." I avoid saying *stillborn*, because I've noticed lately that when I do it makes people respond as though my loss is less. And when that happens, I'm reminded of a study on the experiences of families after the death of their baby, where Dr. Joanne Cacciatore, founder of the MISS Foundation and a bereaved parent herself, refers to our society's frequent belief in the "age commensurate grief myth": that the intensity of mourning increases with the age of the child who died.[3]

Her face softens, and her eyes turn down as she apologizes. I realize it's an apology spoken from a place of understanding when she whispers, "I miscarried when I was two months pregnant. My due date was this fall."

I share the details of Reid's death, and we talk for a little while after we've reached this unwanted common ground. She tells me she hasn't been able to discuss her loss with anyone who's had a similar one before.

I think about how people are often advised against announcing a pregnancy during the first twelve weeks, partly because this is when the risk of miscarriage is the highest. But by making miscarriage private, who does this protect? What if instead we advised people to think about what they might do, or whom they might tell, if miscarriage occurs?

Sometimes it's necessary to take a break from the titles we identify with, and sometimes there's unparalleled beauty in sharing the same identity with another. Something changes when another person is able to validate your pain.

● ☾ ●

ONCE, I BELIEVED in the order of things. I believed my life would follow that order. You were born, and you made it to your late twenties or thirties before your grandparents would die. It would be sad, of course, but they would be good deaths. Natural and expected. Then, once you were in your fifties or sixties, your parents would pass. The world would collapse around you, but you always knew that you would outlive them. It would take a while, but eventually life would carry on. Then, you yourself would return to dust and the cycle would continue—somewhere else, with some other life.

A few years after my high school graduation, a classmate a year younger than me died suddenly at the age of twenty-one. Her parents were boarding a plane to where she was traveling in Europe. She wasn't well, that was all they were told. But as they were en route, she died. The hospital had called her sister, and somehow, the news made it back to me. I ran to the bathroom and was sick. Knowing that her parents were on a plane, probably not knowing yet that their child had died—it seemed too horrible to be real.

Later, her dad began to write on her Facebook wall daily. Every single day he would say something to her.

Love you always daughter

Dad

Even now, he continues to write to her. I remember talking to my mother about it, a year or so after she'd died. "Someone should write to Facebook to have her account deactivated. This isn't healthy," I said. And she agreed, it was painful.

My god, what did I know then about grief? What did either of us know? I wasn't looking out for that father at all; *I* was the problem. I was uncomfortable with his grief. His loss didn't fit with what I understood to be the normal order of things, and his grief reminded me of that.

What I wanted back then was exactly what most people want from me now. To see the grieving happy again, as if grief isn't normal and happy is, and that should be our default setting. To know that somehow, everything always works out. But as I read through her social media, saw the love letters from her grieving father, a small crack appeared in my confidence. Maybe, I thought, just maybe, the workings of this world were more unfamiliar than I'd first assumed. Maybe I'm not so invincible after all.

I am starting to mourn, actively calling grief back into my heart. Two years from now, I'll learn about the difference in Joan Didion's memoir, *The Year of Magical Thinking*, written after the sudden death of her husband and detailing the first year, when she somehow believes that he will come back. In her book, she makes the distinction between grieving and mourning. Grieving, she says, is what happens naturally as a response to the death of a loved one. It is passive. Mourning, by contrast, is something that is consciously done. I see this same idea referenced in Dr. Joanne Cacciatore's study on family experiences of stillbirth, quoting the work of Dr. Scott Eberle: "'Grief is a hardwired feature of human biology... biologically determined' and mourning is socially influenced and culturally determined."[4]

With my days completely occupied by my training I don't have the time to focus on Reid every minute of every day, like I did before. I can't lie in bed for hours and stare at a photo of his perfect face, or journal about our forty weeks together until my hand cramps up.

I wanted to find a new purpose, a new plan, and I had. So why is it that I feel so selfish pursuing it? If Reid were here in my arms as a chubby newborn, I'd be with him all the time. I feel I am cheating him out of our time together. If he were here, I wouldn't be exploring new career paths, I wouldn't be writing nearly as much, I wouldn't have met all these amazing friends who'd also lost children, I wouldn't be training to teach yoga, and I wouldn't have tattooed my firstborn son's name on my wrist. But these are all beautiful, good things, and so I am stuck between feeling like his passing has been the most devastating thing to happen to me and like it is my greatest inspiration. It's what my dad said could happen if I chose to shape my life after loss a certain way, to focus on the good. Still, I'm not sure I'm ready for new dreams. I want the original one.

I wish Reid had a Facebook wall. I imagine what I would write to him:

I love you. I miss your kicks. I hope you're okay.
Mom

● ☾ ●

IN TRAINING, WE are going over *The Yoga Sutras of Patanjali*, texts that cover the philosophy of yoga. From the other side of the circle we are sitting in, someone reads aloud the second sutra, "Yogàs citta vrtti nirodhah." Then they read the translation, "The restraint of the modifications of the mind-stuff is Yoga."

How do I get this kind of power over my mind? During training, it's not so difficult. As I focus on alignment, follow my breath in and out of my body, bring my attention to only what is happening on my mat, everything else gets quiet. The pain of living without Reid is somehow tolerable. And though I feel Reid close in the movements that connect me to my pregnancy, this does not paralyze me. The feeling comes and goes, and I let it. As I study anatomy and interact with the other trainees, a switch is flipped. I can function in this environment where my mind is required to be fully present somewhere outside of my grief.

But then I leave the studio, or we're on a break between modules, or I'm awake in the middle of the night. My brain runs through everything that's happened, in chronological order, and takes dark tangents wherever it pleases. Whether it's torturously looking to relive Reid's death or desperately seeking clarity as to how it got here, I'm not sure.

If I can bring what I'm learning in yoga off my mat and out of that room, I might just survive my grief. I read the sutra again, highlight the end of it, which goes like this:

If you control your mind, you have controlled everything. Then there is nothing in this world to bind you.

I have to go back to the blood lab, the one I had gone to for testing during my pregnancy. Because despite the flying colors I'd received while pregnant with Reid, I'm not passing tests now. I have started to have heart palpitations, notice frequent skipped beats, and I'm not sleeping. I feel as if I need to move, all the time. My body is confused and stressed and completely out of whack. It worked so much better when it was sustaining Reid.

My hair is also finally doing its postpartum thing, and I'm shedding like a golden retriever. Strands a couple of feet long coil around my arms in yoga, leaving piles on my mat. They clog up my drain and accumulate in every corner of my apartment, reminding me how recent my loss is. It doesn't feel that way.

I grieve the loss of that hair, hair that grew with Reid. When it comes out in clumps in the shower I collect it from the bottom of the tub and write his name with it on the shower wall, saying his name aloud as I shape the letters in front of me.

Life feels harder than in the initial months after saying goodbye to Reid. I really don't want to move forward. I want to go back. I want Reid back.

● ☾ ●

OUR LIVES CONTINUE along three different parallels. In the first, we are reliving the months of my pregnancy with Reid, through the #ninemonthswithreid celebrations online. In the second, our world revolves around all the anniversaries of significant dates. In the third—well, that third alternate universe is the one where Reid gets to live. Somewhere out there, there was no knot and no baby died and we get to parent him as we'd always imagined.

And so when the calendar shows July 24, I'm transported into that second world again. On that morning a year ago, I watched the shadows of our bedroom dissolve with the arrival of the sun's early orange light, felt the thick summer breeze enter through the open window and give life to an apartment that didn't yet feel like home, busied myself until the drugstore down the street was open.

I was late, even for me. Although we weren't entirely ready to have kids, Aaron and I weren't using birth control because we knew we wanted them, and my irregular and infrequent cycles hinted that it might be difficult to conceive on our own. We didn't want to miss a rare chance. Each time it was a question, the possibility of having created new life made us feel both terrified and wildly powerful all at once.

This day was no exception. I remember the trip to the drugstore, the bright pink box on the bathroom counter. I remember the tears that flowed when those two solid pink lines appeared. I remember the phone call to Aaron, the sweetness of his excitement on the other end of the line. Mostly, I remember my confidence in the joyous future that test promised: parenthood, a spring baby, a family of our very own.

● ☾ ●

MY YOGA TEACHER training is done; a certificate that sits on my desk says that I'm a qualified instructor. What do I do with this now? Teaching is the obvious answer, but that doesn't feel safe yet. I need to keep learning.

I keep thinking back to Reid's birth and to the people who helped us through it. I think especially of Jill, our doula—the familiar face who calmed us in the depths of pain and exhaustion. How she put her hands on my shoulders, explained what I was going through. How, when my legs wouldn't stop shaking, she told me it was just the hormones. How she took hundreds of photos during it all, and told me she was taking them instead of asking me. At the time, I was convinced I'd never look at them; now I look at them daily. When we first found out Reid had passed away, I wasn't sure I wanted a doula anymore—what was the point? But now I know that it would have been a very different experience without her.

I want to be this person for other families—in life, but mostly in death. I want to support people during one of life's greatest transitions. I want them to know right away that they aren't alone, that this awful thing happens sometimes, that they are not to blame. I want them to know their options. I want them to have the same experience we had, but better. Ultimately, I want to find a way to be there for other families going through the same thing we went through. I know from my conversations with other parents, from my reading, that there's so much room for growth in stillbirth care. And I want to help.

This leads to my decision to register in a doula training program the same week I receive that certificate. This is something to do. To let me feel capable again. In the days since I've graduated, I've been hit hard by a wave of emotions. Everything I suppressed to get through the training finally has time to be felt—and these emotions *demand* it. Tonight, they are debilitating. Aaron has long since retired to the bedroom, but I slither into the nursery, collapse on the glider, and rock back and forth as I study every single photo we have with Reid, of my pregnancy and his birth.

It's been a while since I've really looked at our photos from April 4 and relived the feelings of that day. I told myself I'll never forget those moments—and I won't—but some of them are becoming distorted, bent through the passage of time. There are pockets of time I can't quite recall, and then there are the moments I deliberately imprinted in my mind.

But his birth was only a fraction of our time with him. It's more difficult for me to remember what it was like to be pregnant. I didn't realize that those nine months would be the only months I'd have with him. It was easy to believe that Reid only felt love and that I was calm, relaxed, and happy all the time. But the truth was, I'm only human. I sometimes fell short, as humans do. There were moments when I struggled with the changes in my body, questioned how much I really wanted motherhood, feared what I'd lose more than anticipated what I'd gain. Then, in the moments where the excitement bubbled over, I wanted to rush through to the point where I imagined it would all begin: at birth. I did my best, but I wasn't present nearly as often as I now wish I had been.

I can't leave the nursery tonight, can't abandon the feeling of being near him again. I climb into Reid's crib and cuddle with his stuffed elephants as I stare up at his elephant mobile. There are elephants all over his room—he either would have loved them or been terrified of them. I wind up the mobile and listen to it play "Twinkle, Twinkle, Little Star" as the elephants dance in circles. The next thing I know, it's nearly six AM and the sun is starting to rise. I don't know where I should be, but I have a sense that this isn't it. And still, I watch the morning colors throw light on the sky and get lost in the heartache.

● ☾ ●

THESE DAYS, TIME is not my ally. My idle mind looks for reasons this happened, wanting numbers to explain the stories I've heard that are similar to mine. Even though I stopped seeking comfort in statistics once we joined the "one in" group—those on the wrong side of the statistic—I still need to know: How common is stillbirth *really*?

My research leads me to *The Lancet*, and I learn that we are one of 2.6 million families who have experienced a third-trimester stillbirth in 2015 alone.[5] How was I never aware of this possibility before it became my reality? Can I blame medical advances and societal changes and Western privileges for shielding me from seeing stillbirth as a potential part of life?

Another resource puts this statistic in more digestible numbers. Every day, worldwide, 7,300 people in the last three months of pregnancy will experience the reality of stillbirth.[6] These numbers are not distributed equally: 98 percent occur in low- and middle-income countries, with 77 percent in sub-Saharan Africa and southern Asia. The rate ranges from around three to six stillbirths for every one thousand births in high-income countries like Canada, the US, and the UK, to over forty-three stillbirths per thousand births in Pakistan—the country with the highest reported rates.[7]

I read these numbers over and over again. If these are accurate, why don't we talk about it? It's considered too uncomfortable to discuss socially, but even scientifically, stillbirth remains understudied. One study about stillbirth rates and risk factors in *The Lancet* reveals that less than 5 percent of neonatal deaths and even fewer stillbirths are registered.[8] Comparing statistics from around the world can also be tricky because different countries define stillbirth differently, based on fetal weight, weeks of pregnancy, or other factors.

Another statistic from *The Lancet* reveals that of the 2.6 million yearly stillbirths, "1.2 million of those babies begin labor alive and die before birth," suggesting that many of these deaths are not inevitable. In high-income countries, 20 to 30 percent of stillbirths can be linked to substandard care, and those numbers increase significantly with late-term deaths during birth.[9] And some risk factors for stillbirth can potentially be changed.[10] There's no doubt that even in developed countries, inequality affects birth outcomes. A study that looked at over 15 million pregnancies in the US and UK found that black women are almost twice as likely to experience a stillbirth as white women,[11] and in Canada, Indigenous women have higher rates of stillbirths and other birth complications.[12]

All of this angers me. The numbers are too high. And all of this spurs me to action. We have to talk about stillbirth facts, because there is so much to correct.

Through it all, there is hope. There are people working on research for preventing stillbirth, improving bereavement care, and increasing awareness. In a study in Ireland to gauge the general public's knowledge about stillbirth, over half of those surveyed were unable to identify any risk factors for stillbirth, and less than 1 percent identified reduced fetal movement.[13]

So how much should we educate pregnant people about stillbirth? If not in pregnancy, should it happen before? And how much information is too much? What's the line between scaring parents and potentially preventing a loss?

One study revealed that most women were surprised by stillbirth statistics, and upon learning of them, most agreed that messaging around stillbirth should be subtle, focusing on how to reduce risk and have a safer pregnancy, using positive imagery.[14] Another study, from Australia, about messaging around safe sleep positions in pregnancy, also looked into the benefits and side effects of giving information on risk prevention to pregnant women: Would giving this advice make women anxious? Was this a good or bad thing? To what extent is anxiety in this context beneficial?[15]

And what about the care received after a loss has occurred? It used to be standard to take the baby away immediately after birth before the family could see them. We know now that time spent with the child can be hugely important for families. But not all health care providers know this, nor is the practice applied in any standard way. In an international study about care practices after stillbirth, tremendous inconsistencies in implementation of these practices were discovered.[16] Of the three thousand mothers from high-income countries and six hundred mothers from middle-income countries included in the study, mothers in middle-income countries were less likely to be offered recommended care, such as spending time with their baby, holding them and having family and friends meet them, creating memories with their baby, taking them home, naming them, or organizing a funeral in their honor. But even those from higher-income countries received subpar care.

Then there are the partners—perhaps the most neglected people in the picture. A Canadian study on supporting fathers after stillbirth admitted, "in spite of health professionals' good will, fathers' grief after a stillbirth remains invisible and is barely taken care of by the health services in Canada."[17] Most providers said this was due to a lack of education. The research team that conducted this study has spent fifteen years researching and developing resources, including online videos, books, and workshops, to fill this need. Following stillbirth, fathers or partners have appreciated receiving their own messages of condolence, and have benefited from having an outlet for their grief—physical activity or support groups or one-on-one social situations.

It's important to also look at care specific to pregnancy after stillbirth. In a UK study, a research team developed the Rainbow Clinic at St. Mary's Hospital in Manchester to provide specialized care for pregnancies after stillbirth. Their care plans may include increased monitoring, in an effort to reduce parents' anxiety and to screen for potential problems. Care is usually led by a consistent team of providers, which allows the family to avoid the stress and trauma of having to retell their story at each appointment. They claimed there were no subsequent stillbirths, and that NICU admissions for infants were nearly halved. So should these clinics become standard worldwide?[18]

I don't know that it makes it any easier or more difficult for a parent to know this information, but I believe we have a duty to do the best we can to get it out there, and to improve on it. We shouldn't be silent about stillbirth. *We* as the families experiencing it, as the medical professionals studying it, as the writers able to spotlight it. More research and knowledge and talking about it can only help.

● ☾ ●

IN THE EARLY hours of the morning Reid was born, there was a blood moon, a total lunar eclipse. A magical event when the earth casts its shadow on a full moon and blocks it from the sun, giving it a red glow. When my parents drove to the hospital to meet our firstborn son, their eyes were fixed to the sky to witness the great transformation. It gave the reality of our situation an otherworldly feel that seemed fitting. After all, babies didn't die in the world we lived in.

Since then the moon has always connected me to Reid. Whenever there is a full moon I look into the sky and swear I can feel the weight of his body return to my arms. And when the sun will one day blacken and the moon turn to blood again, I like to think I'll gaze at the rainbow of deep red, rusty orange, pale yellow, grayish blue, and white, and hold on to the hope he gave me.

One evening in August, I keep my sister Alana company while she gets a tattoo. I watch in awe as the needle pierces the surface of her skin over and over for nearly three hours. An artist, she designed the image herself: on one side a stunningly vibrant abstract flower, on the other a mountainscape and full moon, meant to be a tribute to Reid. In the last minutes, the artist starts on the moon—Reid's moon—coloring the spaces between Alana's freckles with white, tracing the symbol of his birth in front of my eyes. When it is finished, Alana sits up and turns her arm to me. My jaw drops. The moon is starting to bleed, painting a circle of red—a blood moon. It is the only part of her tattoo that bled.

In this tattoo parlor, in a part of town on the cusp between trendy and grungy, I am reminded that there is beauty in the unexpected, in this unplanned life after loss. Maybe a willingness to see it is the foundation I need, the thing that will allow me to discover how to keep going. Even though I do not want this life, I still want to live. Don't I?

9

SEPTEMBER FEELS VERY far away from April, and the thought that nearly half a year has passed makes me weep. The third of the month, five months since Reid died, and things don't feel any easier than they did that first month. I have a growing list of all the places I try to avoid:

- Neighborhoods with playgrounds
- Malls with areas for small children to play
- Grocery stores with toddler-sized carts
- The part of town my midwifery clinic is located in
- Coffee shops with toys
- Anywhere I might glimpse a pregnant belly or baby the age Reid would have been

Despite the list, I can't avoid all triggers. When a stranger walks by and brings a waft of Ivory Snow detergent or when someone shouts "Reid!" I wonder if my body will always respond, whether my heart will always quicken, or my body flush with heat, or pools of tears form in the corners of my eyes. I wonder if there will ever come a time when these reminders are welcome.

Despite all of this, well-meaning people tell me I am "coping so well" and "so incredibly strong" and that they "don't know how I do it"—compliments that sound nice but mostly baffle me. I read their words or stare them in the face and wonder what I must look like. What makes me seem strong? Is it the fact that I get up each day or that I plant a smile on my face? Or is it the tears I don't hide or the brokenness that I share?

These words are meant to help, to acknowledge that others see I'm doing the impossible, continuing to live after loss. But I don't *feel* strong. I can't believe that time keeps moving. When I look at the clock and see that seconds, minutes, then hours have gone by, I'm shocked. Every time. As those hours turn into days, and then months, I'm reminded constantly that we didn't just lose Reid; we lost his anticipated presence in all aspects of our lives. I don't think people realize how relentless grief can be. I don't think I realized it either. I have to make a conscious effort every single day to keep going. And at the end of the day, when I can finally slip back under the sheets, I feel depleted, like getting there has taken all the energy in the world. And yet, time keeps moving.

I used to think that strength came from shutting out pain, ignoring emotions. But I learned quickly that it was the opposite. Now I think the strongest people are the ones who let the pain run through their veins—they work with it, feel it. The strongest souls have suffered and are exposed, sensitive, soft.

I feel soft. Reid softened me. My heart, my skin, my body. If I am strong it is only because he opened me up so that I could feel all of the pain in order to survive it. He is the reason I choose to be strong in my vulnerability.

In a world that preys on weakness, I realize it will require tremendous effort to believe in that strength. Vulnerability is not actually a choice. I wonder now if it's a necessary part of being human. What we do with that choice—what we do with that vulnerability—can define how these losses change us. Perhaps it is true that what we think makes us weak is what can actually make us strong.

And on the anniversaries of his death, more than any other days, that vulnerability doesn't look like the coping or strength or functioning that prompt those compliments. As I feel my own body physically unraveling, this feels especially true at month five. These are days I question everything all over again, when I want to disappear, break something, go on a bender, give up. But I can't fade away because I am living for Reid, and sometimes that bothers me too. I want to make him proud (can I still make him proud?), but I wish I didn't have to.

Five months ago my son died inside me, the day before he was due to be born. Why doesn't this sound real yet? Words escape me, but I open up my diary anyway. This is the only thing I manage to write:

It really fucking sucks.
It really fucking sucks.
It really fucking sucks.
Fuck. Fuck. FUCK!

I underline the last *fuck* three times. I immediately feel better, and then embarrassed that something as simple as littering my diary with profanity can make me feel better. What a mess.

● ☾ ●

WHEN I WAS five months pregnant with Reid, just before Christmas last year, I went to the mall with Brittany, pregnant with Charlotte. We roamed through the stores, crossing all the necessary gift purchases off our lists, but our real objective was the candy store. Reid and Charlotte had given both of us a serious sweet tooth, and sour keys were a regular staple for me. Running on sugar, we headed to shop for baby clothes, our hearts melting as we sifted through the impossibly small newborn onesies and talked about the outfits we'd dress our babies in.

Today, on September 4, five months after his birth, we're all back at the mall for #ninemonthswithreid, and I meet Charlotte for the first time. She is loud, like her mama, and has the same big, round eyes and contagious giggle. As she babbles and drinks milk, it is the first time I witness what Reid would have been doing had he lived. I can imagine the movements his body could be making, the space he might have taken up in his car seat, the rolls that may have formed around his knees. I take pleasure in imagining myself placing a five-month-old Reid next to his friend, and then I hear this imaginary self sigh as it remembers this is fantasy. As Brittany and I walk around, eat our candy, drink our smoothies, and talk about our babies, it feels oddly normal.

"Can I hold her?" I ask Brittany, surprising myself with the request.

"Oh, Emma," she replies, eyes turning red around the rims. "Absolutely."

I hold my arms out and am startled by the weight of her. Immediately, Charlotte reaches to grab my hair and a few strands catch between her sticky fingers. Brittany helps me untangle from her grasp, and Charlotte is grinning with pride.

Holding her brings home that she isn't Reid, and seeing her beam up at me makes it impossible to be upset.

We go back to the candy store and put his five-month tie sticker on the sour key jar, just for a moment to take a picture, and as we are snapping away, a beautiful thing happens: Charlotte puts her hand on the sticker, strokes it, and smiles. The feeling that follows, so like joy, is unexpected. Maybe I'm realizing there is no scenario for the present where Reid is here with us. I can imagine it—that perfect plan I kept so close—but it was a dream.

I think back to when Amy visited last month, when I saw her for the first time since Reid passed away. I wasn't ready to meet her daughter, so her husband, David, walked her around the neighborhood as we talked.

"I don't want to rush this," she said. "But I want to let you know now that I will need to leave in about two hours to nurse Grace."

"Of course," I replied, walking back to where she was sitting on our couch. I looked at her and couldn't help but notice how swollen her breasts were with milk. I pictured what her daughter must look like at her chest. I remembered what it was like for our bellies to grow together. I thought of the many hours of conversations we had about our kids growing old together. I tried to fight back tears, and I failed.

Then Amy was crying, too. I was afraid of that. And yet, even though my fears were realized, it felt right to be raw and open and honest. It hurt like hell to be reminded of all that was and that should have been, but it also felt normal. It felt healing to sit and cry tears of pain and joy with my friend. We were still both postpartum mothers. And it felt so good to talk about our babies as we emptied yet another box of tissues. We sat on the couch and we cried, and cried, and cried. The tears that open us are some of the sweetest.

These friends, their own birth stories, and their present motherhood experiences, are both interlaced with mine. They have their own grief, and they acknowledge mine. They send texts to let me know the little ways they are reminded of Reid. (*His name was mentioned while I was out today. It made me happy to hear it.*) They let me know they're thinking of him, even though I don't usually respond. (*I am awake with a screaming baby right now. I just wanted to say that I am thinking of you and how you're probably up as well, but not with Reid. I am crying for you, Emma. I miss him too.*)

I miss Reid. I miss the place he could have occupied in our lives. As the months go on and Reid's friends continue to grow, it will always be hard to not see him here growing with them. And though it doesn't always feel like it, others are missing him too. It's easy to identify in these moments of connection.

I think it's hard for friends of a grieving parent to know how to give comfort, or if they should. It's hard to step in and it's hard to do nothing, to find normalcy in a situation that is far from normal.

Micaela and Hanah have started to avoid talking about their problems. When they would share the usual complaints—work was long, a friend was rude—I would nod and say, "Ah yes, how awful," but the words tasted sour in my mouth. I don't have the patience or the heart for these conversations anymore, and I think they can tell. Eventually the sharing dwindles. I'm being a terrible friend, but they keep showing up for me, and I vow that one day, when I've made it through the intense season of early grief, I will show up for them again. I don't know how long it will be before I'm able to ask about their love lives or jobs. Or how much longer after that when I will actually care to hear the answer.

I make new friends over shared heartaches, friendships that exist both online and in person. Women who have lost children too and are able to hold space for Reid in our conversations. They ask questions I didn't know I needed to be asked: Was his skin very fragile? Was he warm on my chest? Were his fingernails long? They ask to see photos and simply nod when I confess the smallest and darkest of details.

These new friendships grate on some old ones, I think. Some friends, who don't understand the way I'm choosing to grieve, operate out of anger and judgment. I can't fault them for this. I think they're grieving their own loss, because the Emma they knew, the friend they had in me, is gone. I will wonder later if the chaos and heartache and unpredictable nature of what passed between me and some friends was because of this, because they were grieving too. They wanted to go back to a relationship that didn't exist anymore.

I've given myself permission to accept the secondary losses of friendships now, learned how to integrate these losses and move forward. I can't pretend to be who I no longer am to preserve them. Grief can both shatter the old and bind the new in the most unexpected ways when it comes to human connections. There's no one to blame or credit; that's simply how it is.

● ☾ ●

WE ARE PAST the halfway point of celebrating the forty weeks of my pregnancy. I can't think about what might happen when we've had more time missing Reid than time spent with him. I leave that thought unturned.

Today is another day belonging to that second parallel world that revolves around the anniversaries of our time with Reid. September 17, the date I will forever remember as the day we shared our pregnancy with the world on social media. We wrote *Mom* and *Dad* on coffee cups and held them out in front of our faces toward the camera. The decaf box was checked off on mine and the number three was scribbled on Aaron's—surely, living with a pregnant me would require lots of caffeine.

I wonder now why we did it that way. As I stare at those cups that live on our bookshelf, I wonder: Did we really feel we were already parents? As we discovered his personality, fretted at his doctor's appointments, documented his milestones, and loved him with all we had, did we feel we were already well into our roles as mom and dad? Did we realize that we would consider him our first child, no matter what?

I can't remember—or I don't want to. So much has changed in the year since that announcement, but we are always Mom and Dad.

●	☾	●

I'M STILL RELIVING the day Reid was born. Playing it backward and forward, pausing when I want to stay in a moment, and fast-forwarding when a memory is too much to bear. I'm beginning to remember more of the little things. How I instinctively placed my palm against Reid's belly as Aaron cut the cord, making sure he didn't scratch his delicate skin. How I kept apologizing to his mortal body, over and over again: *I'm so sorry, baby. I'm so sorry.* The sound of my makeup hitting the bathroom floor as I scrambled to make myself presentable for his portraits, not wanting to be away from his side for a minute. The way his hat kept slipping off his head.

I spend an untold number of hours looking for an explanation that will take away the pain I'm feeling. I've always been uncomfortable with pain, preferring to put a neat and tidy bow on whatever I can, to fix things that break.

When I was growing up, my parents made sure everyday worries and struggles were never ours. My childhood was a truly happy one. Yes, I knew vaguely that something terrible had happened to my father when he lost the use of his legs, but when I arrived in this world, nearly two decades after his accident, he'd done an amazing thing with his situation. I never witnessed the grief and struggle to get there, never saw the choices that had to be made to head in that direction.

I understood this to mean that if you worked hard enough, things would always turn out alright.

As I got older I was able to appreciate my privilege for the foundation it gave me, and I'm grateful for the protection I had. But did this prepare me for the inevitable hardships I would experience?

When I was nineteen and living in London, I got a call from my father saying that my mother was in the hospital and would have a procedure done on her heart in a few days' time. I was silent on the other end of the line. She'll be fine, he assured me. No need to come home. So I didn't, not right away.

It wasn't until I sat in the doctor's office years later, twenty weeks pregnant with Reid, when we were going through my family's medical history, that I heard it for the first time. "So," she began, scrolling through my file, "your mom had a heart attack before age fifty?" She shook her head, clearly surprised.

I mumbled a few noises, trying to fake a composed confirmation. But it was news to me. There had been talk of chest pain, clogged arteries, and stents, sure. But a heart attack? Never. I once thought that bad things didn't happen to us, but I wonder if the truth is simply that we didn't mention them.

While my father remains my compass for navigating trials, and we talk often about our different life-altering experiences, I am unprepared for the road ahead. I stumble between good days and terrible days. And in my travels I wander closer to God.

I haven't been able to stop writing about the feeling that God has been so near to me. I've never felt anything like what I felt in that hospital giving birth to Reid, never felt less alone than when I left him there in that nurse's arms, never felt so broken but so held in my entire life. I can't stop attacking this feeling from every possible angle, talking and blogging about it. It's out of character for me. Whenever I've talked of religion in the past, I preferred to reference text and literature and theology over feelings. That I've been recounting the story of my own sensations of something supernatural has me puzzled. I share it anyway.

But the feeling is fading now. I have this inkling that I'm slowly being deserted. So I pick up the Bible, I listen to sermons online, I devour books by well-known pastors. All the while, I become more aware of my inability to reconcile that the God I'm learning more about could have allowed my son to die, but also filled me with such love in the process. Maybe all of this can be chalked up to the light, numbing sensation of protection that shock offers, followed by its wearing off. If I'm looking at this logically, both options are possible.

Later, I will read Kate Bowler's memoir and something she says will bring me back to this feeling. An associate professor at Duke Divinity School, she writes about her life and faith relating to her terminal cancer diagnosis, but there is one passage that I keep coming back to. Right after receiving her cancer diagnosis, when she isn't sure she will survive the year, she talks about the incredible sensation that God is near, that she is filled with love. She writes:

> *That feeling stayed with me for months. In fact, I had grown so accustomed to that floating feeling that I started to panic at the prospect of losing it. So I began to ask friends, theologians,*

historians, pastors I knew, and nuns I liked, What am I going to do when it's gone? *And they knew exactly what I meant because they had either felt it themselves or read about it in great works of Christian theology. St. Augustine called it "the sweetness." Thomas Aquinas called it something mystical like "the prophetic light." But all said yes, it will go. The feelings go. The sense of God's presence will go. There will be no lasting proof that God exists. There will be no formula for how to get it back.*

And this is it exactly. This feeling that overwhelmed me in the hospital with Reid—I could only describe it as feeling God near. Though I didn't have a near-death experience, I carried death inside me. It took place as Reid and I were connected. I consider it possible that our connection allowed for some transference of this experience of grace.

In all my suffering and questioning and wondering, He was right there. Will He ever be a God that I fully understand? Will I find the answers I long for in my searching? Do I trust this God to want to hear them? The only question I can answer right now is the last one. I do trust Him. It's easy, really. I have to. Because with Him there is hope that I'll see Reid again.

I also want to know more about this transition that Reid has endured. I've never given much serious thought to what this reunion might be like, but after reading Meghan O'Rourke's words in *The Long Goodbye* I do for the first time. Writing after the loss of her mother, she said:

Believing in heaven doesn't protect you from the intensities of grief. To contemplate death in any serious way, even as a believer, is to wonder what change death wreaks upon us. In the occasional moments when I believe in forces we cannot see, I still find it impossible to believe in the cinematic image of loved ones waiting for me just like normal—if slightly diaphanous and shimmering—as I cross a river into their yearning embrace. It simply does not make sense that so enormous a transition would lead to so similar an existence.

Even though I believe in heaven, I still fight the notion of meeting Reid there. I still grieve. Passages from the Bible suggest that we will be different in heaven—better, whatever that means. But if I'm being entirely honest, I don't want better. I want what I had when the child I loved was alive, the treasured flesh and blood that kicked and rolled.

What would it be like to meet again? When I think of it, I don't imagine him as an infant. I don't imagine him older either, or in any human form at all, for that matter. He is simply there, and we are together. If it can't happen here, in this form, I hold on to hope that it will happen there, in the unknown. *Together* seems like a blissful state to reach.

● ☾ ●

I'M INCREASINGLY PARANOID about my health. My heart continues to quicken with palpitations, skip beats. There's a spot on my leg; could it be skin cancer? I visit my doctor, who reassures me that the pauses in my heartbeat rhythms are normal responses to changes in blood flow in my body, that the dark spot is not cancerous.

"But what about the extreme hair loss? The inability to sleep but the lack of energy to attempt anything else?" I ask.

"All normal, all to be expected with anyone during the postpartum period," she answers.

But this doesn't feel normal.

There's another full moon approaching tonight, September 27, the last of the tetrad of blood moons that Reid's belonged to. I plan to watch it with Aaron on top of a mountain. The next blood moon is three years away, and the next supermoon/ blood moon combo won't be until 2033. It's incredible and wonderful and so very lucky that we will always have such a specific reminder of Reid's birth and the last few hours we had with him. Not a reminder that consumes us every day, or even every year, but a big, beautiful reminder that will grace us with its appearance every now and then, perhaps right at the moments we need it.

I'm making my way through my doula training. I finished the course and have started to read the textbooks required for certification. And now I am working alongside a mentor doula to gain real-life experience. We attended a prenatal visit together a couple of weeks ago, and I've been on call for the family's birth ever since. I'm nervous.

As fate would have it, our client's waters broke this morning. So I know that instead of sitting on a mountain with Aaron, I'll be back at the hospital, back where I was under another blood moon, birthing my own babe into the world, but this time helping another brave family bring theirs here too.

A text from the senior doula I'm training with says she's on her way to the hospital and I should get there as soon as possible. I scramble to put together some food and start to make a pot of coffee, then quickly remember that coffee is one of those scents that could set off a person in labor. Instead, I boil water for tea and throw two bags of lavender Earl Grey into a tumbler.

As I pull into the parking lot and turn the engine off I stare at the giant hospital sign before me. Memories of Reid wash over me, and I feel raw and exposed. But feeling that much nearer to my son also gives me the courage I'll need to make it through the birth. If I close my eyes, I can even picture his face in the crook of my arm again.

I walk toward the entrance. One foot. Then the next. Not quite knowing what to expect, or how I'll feel. But as soon as I walk through those doors, I'm there for that family, to support Natalie and Vince in their experience of birthing their child. I'm not there to relive my own experience. A blood moon is an omen for a big change, I know. Maybe this is a reminder to honor my vow: to cherish my memories with Reid while living confidently in the present.

I'm standing at Natalie's feet when the head finally emerges. The bright light of the obstetrician's station points directly at it and my breath fills every crevice of my lungs. The baby is caught between two worlds. One more push and they'll leave the only world they've ever known and be thrust into this wild one that makes little sense but is so beautiful. In this moment, the difference between birth and death doesn't seem so big.

The next morning I wake to warmth between my thighs. I shift slightly and catch the familiar scent of rust. Quietly, I waddle to the bathroom and watch a flood of crimson fill the toilet bowl beneath me.

IO

THE FIRST TIME we discussed wanting to conceive again, Reid's body was still warm in my arms. I lay propped up in the hospital bed, the epidural flowing through me, Aaron sitting to my left. The sky was dark in the window above him. Through quiet sobs he told me, "I want this," as he traced the roundness of Reid's cheeks. "I want this so badly."

I knew exactly what he meant. "I do too," I said, turning toward him and watching the tears fall in a steady stream off the edge of his jaw.

"Let's get pregnant again quickly," he said.

I nodded. "Yes."

It might be hard to understand that we could think of a second baby so soon after losing our first. The feeling was primal, a decision made for us. As my body went through all its postpartum motions—the slow and steady bleeding of a healing womb, the milk leaking from expectant breasts, the insomnia meant to mimic a newborn cycle—the possibility of creating new life that it could one day sustain became a sort of balm for the rawness of it all. It was the only idea that could temper the sting of acute grief, if only for brief moments at a time. For each tear we cried for our son, we cried another tear for our future as parents to him.

I don't always understand it. I just know that it feels like the only way forward. And I know that when we actively started trying again, after being cleared at the six-week mark, it wasn't an act of trying to replace Reid in any way, because he will never be replaced. Children aren't interchangeable. Another child won't ever fill the hole that Reid has left. But aside from getting Reid back, only another baby can bring us any true happiness. We want a sibling for Reid. Another child might fill our broken hearts in a different way, but they will never be whole in the same way again. And I don't even want that, because where would that leave Reid?

Within days of Reid's death people started telling me, "You can try again." Some even offered it with their initial condolences: "I'm sorry for your loss. But you'll have another baby." That's exactly what we want, but it doesn't matter. To hear it from others feels like I'm being handed a prescription, as if this is a simple malady, and with the right dose of this or that it can be fixed. "I know how to make this right," these people seem to say. "I recommend another baby within the year and that fickle grief should disappear." I want the baby, but I want to be able to grieve too.

Other times, people seem to want to minimize my loss by comparison. A woman looks me in the eye one day and says, "At least you can have another child. A friend of mine had a miscarriage, then endured five years of infertility only to never conceive again." My heart breaks for her friend, and at the same time, I'm upset by her response. She only wanted to help me, but she just made me feel awful. She turned grief into a contest that I was losing, but it's not one I want to win either. I don't want to play the game at all.

Why compare my unique experience of loss to someone else's? Why do we have this instinct to categorize different situations as more or less than? I just want to let this woman's loss be significant to her, and let mine remain significant to me. We can connect on this common ground without ranking our losses in the process. My life-shattering moment is different from another's and we can still meet each other right where we are.

I understand that people find it difficult to witness others in pain, that it's human to want to help somehow, take it away. But the most helpful thing anyone ever says to me is, "I'm so sorry. I have no idea what you're going through, but this really fucking sucks." No trying to explain the ache away, no trying to overcome grief, no promising that silver linings will be found. But even if the words aren't perfect, that they come from a place of love means the most of all.

● ☾ ●

WE'VE JUST SAT down to Thanksgiving dinner when my phone buzzes. It's my mentor doula, texting to tell me our next client's waters have broken. I know that within the next twenty-four hours the baby will come out, so I turn down wine and clear my schedule for the next two days.

Later that night I get another call. There are signs of meconium and the parents are heading to the hospital. I should get ready to go.

When I show up, my mentor has our client, Veronica, dancing down the halls, hips shaking, trying to get the baby to move on down. Monitors are hooked up to her round belly, and they are showing that the contractions are still irregular. In both of the births I've attended now, the birthing people have been monitored for their entire labors. With each hip sway or trip to the bathroom, the monitors slip and lose the baby's heartbeat and the alarms sound.

The first few times it happened I felt sick to my stomach. I was brought right back to the alarms that were sounding when I found out Reid had passed away. In those moments, it required all my strength to stay in the present. I expect to see a team of doctors and nurses rush in with a portable ultrasound and reveal the worst. But I am starting to realize that this is normal. Monitors slip and sometimes the alarms sound. It doesn't mean a baby has died.

The doctors say they will need to start Pitocin soon to accelerate the labor—the twenty-four-hour mark is fast approaching. I press Veronica's hips together and run firm fingers down the length of her back at each new rush. She moans and sways and closes her eyes tightly. Paul, her partner, walks into the room with a steaming cup of coffee and I chuckle to myself, knowing what will likely soon follow.

"No!" Veronica shouts. "No coffee!" Flustered, Paul looks to us. We tell him to enjoy the coffee in the waiting area and come back after. We have mints in our bags for him when he's done.

When Paul returns, ready to jump back in, I go for a bathroom break. I pull down my pants and immediately see the bright-red blood. The bleeding that appeared after the first birth I attended—just over two weeks ago—has continued, but it was finally starting to taper. Now it is back in full force. My heart sinks. I make a note in my phone to call my doctor when her office opens in the morning, then fish a pad out of my backpack, and resolve not to think about what it might indicate about my health.

Veronica has been laboring hard for about ten hours when the first signs appear that the baby is in distress. The doctor takes a small sample from the skull to test lactate levels, which are high, but not alarmingly so. The family is told that labor can continue for another hour, max, or else they can arrange for their baby to be delivered by cesarean now. Veronica bursts into tears and is shaking from fever and lack of sleep. I want to wrap her up in my arms and stroke her hair as I whisper that everything will be fine. But I can't promise her that. Instead, I silently pray that both she and the baby will make it, rubbing her feet as I do.

We ask the doctors and nurses to leave so that the family can talk about what to do. After my mentor helps them to understand the medical side of things, they decide that they want the baby out safely, and if that means surgery, that's what they will do. An obstetrician is immediately paged and an OR is booked—there's only space for my mentor. I will miss the birth, but I don't care. The baby will be okay. The mother will be okay. They have to be.

I sit outside the operating room, watching surgeons and nurses rush by in their blue and green scrubs, and wait for

Veronica to be wheeled in. Paul and my mentor appear, then quickly leave to change into their own scrubs. Then, Dr. G., my new obstetrician, turns up. She will be doing the C-section.

She sits down next to me and asks me how I am doing—a mini-appointment of sorts. She knows how difficult it is for me to get in to see her, given that she also runs the obstetrics department at the hospital. I explain everything. I'd gotten the results of some of the tests she'd recently run on me, and I pull them up on my phone.

"Oh no," she says, zooming in on a number. "That's too low."

"What is?"

"Your thyroid-stimulating hormone—your TSH—is far below the lower limit," she explains. She tells me this is likely because my thyroid is hyperactive. "Look," she points. "Your free T4 is very high. This could all cause symptoms including heart palpitations, insomnia—"

"Those are all things I'm experiencing," I interrupt. "Why is this happening?"

"It could be postpartum thyroiditis," she says. "But I'll need to run some more tests."

I tell her I'm on day fifteen of my period. "What if it never stops?"

"It will stop. But if it doesn't, call me. And if it gets worse, go to the hospital." She pats the bench between us as if to solidify the plan and takes off to the surgery.

In the end, a healthy baby is born via cesarean. I have been a doula for two families now, and as much as I worried about whether I could separate my own experience from theirs, I'm discovering that it isn't so hard to compartmentalize. Birth is so very different with a living baby, though I still have to overcome some big fears to get through it.

Mostly, I'm in awe of the strength people possess during birth. I truly believe that birth is beautiful in all of its forms—that however a birthing person brings a child earth-side is sacred, because ultimately what matters is that they feel empowered, are healthy, and that the baby is safe. With the tight squeeze of a hand and the release of a moan they endure contraction after contraction after contraction. With shaking limbs and a circle of medical professionals above them they endure the cut, separation, and pull of flesh. They endure it all out of necessity or determination or love. They endure incredible pain and make enormous sacrifices to birth these babies into longing arms. What a wonder.

● ☾ ●

ON HALLOWEEN THE blood is gushing—it feels satirically appropriate, somehow. It's day thirty-three of the never-ending period, and so Aaron and I make our way to the hospital. I feel ridiculous, going to Emergency for a period. The waiting room is packed full of bodies in various conditions of discomfort, from broken limbs to pale faces. I immediately feel guilty for taking time away from them.

The admitting nurse takes us into a cubicle to get our history. I start to recount the facts, beginning with Reid.

"Oh!" she shouts before I'm done talking. "I think I know who you are!" She peers up from her computer. "You're the couple whose birth story went viral, right? I saw it on the news."

"Yes," I say. "That was us."

She offers her condolences, in a polite and professional way, then asks me a series of questions. "Could the bleeding be a miscarriage?" she wonders. And, "Are you sure it's lasted thirty-three days?"

"I don't think it's a miscarriage," I respond. "And I'm sure, it's been thirty-three days."

After admitting, I'm examined and scheduled for tests and a pelvic and transabdominal ultrasound. When I take out my tampon, after the tech leaves the room, blood gushes out of me and hits the floor. Large clots speckle the polished concrete. I frantically run to the paper-towel dispenser on the wall, holding the paper sheet between my legs as I crouch down to wipe the ground clean.

The doctor looks at the results immediately after the ultrasound. There is fluid in my fallopian tubes, which is abnormal, but likely because of how much I'm bleeding. I notice the look on the doctor's face change from sympathetic and disbelieving to sympathetic and curious.

No one ever mentions that every one of the health issues I'm experiencing might be because of grief. In fact, it won't be until I read Joan Didion's *The Year of Magical Thinking* that I first hear that grief can manifest in physiological disruptions. Didion quotes the Institute of Medicine as saying that grief can cause "changes in the endocrine, immune, autonomic nervous, and cardiovascular systems." She herself experienced these changes at New York Hospital on the night her husband died. When remembering how cold she'd felt, she said, "I was also cold because nothing in my body was working as it should."

Is this true? Is there really a physiology to grief? And if so, why did no one tell me?

My body doesn't need any telling; it is simply acting out my grief, showing me that my heart is breaking. The doctor mentions that a diagnosis of postpartum thyroiditis is highly likely. It begins with an overactive thyroid but usually ends up as hypothyroidism, an underactive thyroid. They don't connect it to the bleeding. They don't connect anything to the grief. No matter; I won't be allowed to continue trying to conceive, they say. It's too dangerous for me and for any potential baby. My body has actually become the hazard I felt it was in the weeks after Reid's death.

The doctor gives me two options. The first: take tranexamic acid, which is intense but will stop the bleeding within twenty-four hours. The second: go on the pill to control my cycles while my thyroid goes through the stages of postpartum thyroiditis, then come off it when they can treat it in the hypothyroid stage.

I know that this second option will delay our ability to conceive even further, and I fear for the way my body will respond. Birth control and I have a history. I initially went on it in my teens to regulate my cycles, but when I stopped taking it in my twenties, it took me nearly two years and two rounds of hormone therapy to get my cycles back. I don't know how I would make it through that again, not now.

So I take the tranexamic acid. Almost immediately, it causes my bleeding to intensify. So I end up on birth control anyway. And when that doesn't work, a double dose of it.

For the next few days I'm a self-pitying mess: I'm taking medication I fear and I'm exhausted from a combination of hyperthyroidism-induced insomnia and blood loss. I wander down a rabbit hole of negative scenarios, wallowing in the pit of dark imaginings. *I will never stop bleeding. I will have to stay on the pill forever. I'll probably have to have my uterus removed too. We can never afford adoption. I'll never have another child. This is it.*

Aaron makes sure I have food to eat, a fresh pair of PJs to throw on, a clean shirt to cry into. I don't know much at this point, except that I can't do even these most basic of things without him. Our relationship has had moments where it has faltered and places where it has changed, but we unite in our shared imaginings of parenthood, this obsessive desire strengthening us.

Last month we went on a hike together. We drove to the North Shore and threw on some more layers when the air was cooler than we expected.

"Are there always so many babies on this trail?" I huffed between steps, watching infants strapped to their parents pass us by.

Aaron took my hand and said, "Just follow me."

And I did. I kept my eyes down, tried to match his steps. A mostly impossible task, him being six foot six. The effort of it kept me occupied, though.

We eventually made it to the top, finding a tuft of moss to sit on away from the crowd taking selfies in front of the view.

"Hey," he said.

"Yeah?" I leaned my head on his shoulder.

"We'll be up here with our kid one day."

That he shared my wondering, that he admitted it, was a note of affection. My eyes continued to wander over to the families with small children in that crowd, hoping that what Aaron said was true.

●　◐　●

AFTER FORTY-ONE DAYS, the bleeding stops. I'm nauseous and have piercing headaches, but I need to believe it is over.

I keep telling myself that all of this is happening for a reason. It has to be. Otherwise isn't it all just randomness and chaos with no room for hope? Otherwise do decidedly bad things happen to generally good people for no reason at all? Isn't that worse than believing there is some purpose for suffering? I need to trust that one day, years from now, I will be able to look back on everything that has happened and understand why. It won't change anything about my past, but it could change my present, give me some semblance of order and control.

But in the same way that I don't want promises of healing through new babies, I don't want someone else to tell me that there is a reason my firstborn son died. I need to arrive at my beliefs on my own terms. When those beliefs are projected on me, I can't think clearly.

Still, I cling to the possibility that clarity will come. It is my one redeeming thought. *This is all for a reason. This is all for a reason. This is all for a reason.*

II

N NOVEMBER MY grief is at its worst. Most days I am inconsolable, lying in bed and not moving for anything but food and water. Aaron is by my side when he can be, holding me, absorbing the blows of my violent sobs. I am completely lost. The energy I've poured into distractions and training courses and work has worn thin. I kept busy because I needed to do something, anything, other than mourn. And also because I truly believed that if I just focused on something other than getting pregnant again I would.

Maybe I am wasting my youth. One of my blog readers says as much. They tell me I am wasting the best years of my life in doctors' offices. I can't argue with them, however misguided their motives are. Since Reid's death, it feels like I'm always at a GP or OB or REI or some other arrangement of the alphabet.

When Aaron asks what he can do to help, all I can say is that there is nothing that will help except for the obvious. All

I want is a chance to birth a living child. But with the doctors saying it isn't safe and forbidding me from trying, with the end date of this ban unknown, little can comfort me. Even though I know this will eventually end, I am stuck inside my own pain.

I wonder aloud to Aaron: "What is the point?"

"The point to what?"

When I don't answer he bites his lip and says, "I don't like hearing you say that. Do you really feel like there's nothing to live for right now?"

I take a deep breath. I try to explain it in a way that doesn't make it sound like he isn't enough, when in reality that is exactly the problem. I love Aaron to no end, but is he enough to keep me tethered to the world I no longer want any part of? When my only son has moved on to the next without me?

I assure him that I would never end my own life. Not when I get to live it and my son doesn't. Not while I'm still selfish enough to desire to create and grow and raise another life.

The problem is knowing that Reid is waiting for me elsewhere, and that it wouldn't take much to join him. What makes a life worth living? And by that same token, what makes it worth leaving that life? These are questions I can't answer, and so I do nothing except wail into the night and let my tears stain my husband's shirts. I have the extraordinary feeling of living life with one foot in this world and the other in the next. I ache desperately for the day I will go, when I can finally hold my child again.

There is never a grand attempt. It isn't so irrational to think about, but I'm not thinking with intent, or for attention. I am simply thinking. About death and what my life can withstand before I reach it. I don't know if anything about my grief is ordinary, but it seems natural to explore what it would mean to join the loved one you've lost. To let yourself feel, even when it hurts, even when it scares you—or maybe what I mean is *especially* when.

My family holds a kind of intervention. They sit down around the dinner table at my parents' home one night when I'm over to visit. "We can't stand to see you this miserable. Please let us help," Rebecca says.

"Even when you're here, you're not really here," my mother adds.

"You can't help," I say. "The only thing that can give me hope is the ability to try for another baby. You can't give me that, so there's really nothing to do."

"There has to be something else," my dad says. Some of them are starting to cry now. Their crying makes me feel worse—I can't take on their grief too.

"You have to let me stay sad for a while."

I leave in a huff, not turning back to look at their faces. In the car I text Aaron:

You'll never guess what just happened.

Up until now I've barely even had a glass of wine. I'm hyper-aware that had Reid lived I would be caring for a baby and not drinking excessively, that I could be breastfeeding now. The idea of drowning my grief in alcohol hasn't seemed all that intriguing anyway; I'm already emotional enough.

Besides that, I've been trying to stay healthy. Conceiving is always on my mind. If I get pregnant again, I want my body to be in the best shape possible. But now that I am on birth control—and a double dose—everything has changed. Precisely because nothing is going to change right now. No pregnancy means no potential for a living baby and so my mind sings a different tune: *Fuck it. Why not?*

I go over to Micaela's to spend the evening with her and Hanah. They don't comment on my mood, or try to change it. They rearrange themselves on the couch and make space for me, and for a little while we sit in a silence that's not at all awkward.

We watch a safe, mindless, baby-free chick flick and eat sushi out of takeout containers. Our glasses stay topped up with cool white wine. And I try not to resist how nice it feels to enjoy a simple evening with them.

At the end of the night, sober enough to drive but with a lingering buzz from the liquor, I find myself at a 7-Eleven buying a pack of cigarettes and one pink-and-white polka-dot lighter. The last time I did this I was seventeen and sneaking into a dodgy convenience store that didn't check IDs. I'm shocked at the price: sixteen dollars. How can people afford to smoke regularly?

I drive a few blocks to a wide, open park, get out of the car, and sit down on a bench. I light the cigarette and take three long, slow inhales, gazing at the starry skies. Then I watch the rest of it burn, cringing slightly, as I always do now at the sight of anything burning.

I put it out on the sole of my shoe, chuck it into the city garbage bin, and start my drive home. But then my head starts to fill with anxiety. Maybe the cigarette will set the garbage on fire, maybe security cameras will catch it all, maybe

I'll be arrested, and then I'll go to jail and never have another chance to get pregnant again. It doesn't matter that I clearly put it out.

I do a U-turn, stop in front of the garbage can, put on my hazards, and jump out of the car. I gaze in and see nothing. Still unable to quiet the fear, I walk back to my car to grab my water bottle and return to dump its contents into the bin. *There. That will do it.* Then I burst into a fit of giggles, alone in the middle of a dark city park in the early-morning hours. I have to laugh at myself; I can't even rebel anymore.

When I crawl into bed, and Aaron draws me close, gently parting my lips, I wonder if he can taste the smoke, the familiar taste of ash muddled with flesh. When we were teenagers, we would sometimes buy Zig-Zags and roll our own cigarettes at my family's cabin on the ocean, choosing one night to smoke them as we talked through our hopes and heartaches and dreams for our futures. Rare indulgences of rebellion against our health at a time when we felt we were invincible. It's been a long time since we were those people.

● ☾ ●

I'M SPENDING A LOT of time reading about death. I'm also spending an abnormal amount of time thinking about death. I feel like our family tree is losing branches much too quickly and I fear more will fall.

My mind is braced for trauma, fueled by fear. Bad things happen in threes—isn't that what they say? What will be next? Or *who*? First it was Reid, then my grandpa Marvin in the summer. He had dementia, but pneumonia killed him in the end. I often hear people talk about *good deaths* and *bad deaths*. Reid's, by most criteria, was a "bad death"—sudden and too soon. My grandpa Marvin, by contrast, had a "good death." He lived a relatively long life and illness entered the picture only during his last years. The phrase "He's in a better place" almost worked in his situation. Almost. But attempting to categorize loss can't relieve what is troubling me: that I know I am at risk for further heartbreak.

I think of the imminent deaths in my future. I know they will come, and yet it doesn't seem possible that there could be more. Where I am feels like rock bottom, and the hope that I won't fall any farther grounds me. I am surviving here.

I am not a master of death, deciding who it will take, but I will try to conquer it anyway, and hope that knowledge will somehow keep it away.

On December 5, I get a text from my mom. Her dad, my grandpa Patrick Reid, is in the hospital. It reads:

Grandpa had a massive heart attack this morning. He isn't doing well. They think this is it and are focusing on comfort instead of performing any extreme measures to save him.

A few hours later I text her back and ask how he is doing.

He's gone, she replies.

I call her and we both cry quietly into the phone. All I can think about is the last time I saw him in person, just a few weeks ago at his home. The whole family sat in the living room and discussed his funeral. It wasn't that he was exceptionally unwell, he was just getting older. It seemed morbid to discuss it so openly with him in the room. Although, given that he was the one person who should have any say in the matter, it made sense.

"I want to go out the same way I came in," he kept repeating. "No fuss." And he said it until each of us promised there would be no funeral.

I asked him if we could have some sort of gathering.

"Sure." He sighed. "You can have a little party for me."

"Okay," I replied. "One with a lot of Guinness?"

He nodded and smiled. "Yes, fine."

I sit on the couch and cry into the pillows until there are no more tears. A lifetime without loss and then suddenly so much. But this one feels different. My grandpa Patrick was a part of every milestone of my life, and this is my first experience of losing someone I have a lifetime of intimate memories with. I grew up with my grandpa in the wings for each one of my firsts. From my first day in this world and my first steps to my first love and my marriage.

Most cherished in my memory is the moment we announced our pregnancy. I handed my grandma the ultrasound photo, and after studying it for a moment, she brought her hand up to the side of her face and cried, "You're pregnant!" My grandpa yelled, "I'm going to make it!" and shot his arms straight up into the air. I'd never seen him so uninhibitedly excited. He always said he wouldn't die until he had a great-grandchild. I will always feel a deep sadness that he never got to meet Reid, his namesake, in this life, and a deep comfort at the thought that he was greeted by Reid in the other.

I think of the long and impressive list of his accomplishments and let these soften the grief. Though devastating, his death is natural, timely, follows a life fully lived. And when I read about the Second World War he served in, or hear about Expo 86, which he was commissioner general of, or look at the Canadian flag he had a role in designing, I will think of him. There are reminders of him everywhere, and long after he is gone I will still expect to see him some days. I'll walk into the home he shared with my grandma and imagine he is sitting on the couch around the corner.

I never got this kind of grief with Reid. After losing him, I had no barometer for what I was experiencing. In the beginning, I read endless memoirs and books on loss, and all of them spoke about the phantom-ness that comes after the death of a loved one, but they were mostly about older children or parents or lovers. One would marvel, "But surely, he'll be back. I keep telling myself he's only out for a drive." Or another would weep, "Isn't she just at work?"

These grievers had a presence they could pin to an absence. But Reid was neither here nor there. What I knew of him was attached to me and me alone, except for those few hours in the hospital. I couldn't say, "He's only in the nursery." Because I had no memories of him there.

Instead, I remembered moments from my pregnancy. As I walked by the open door of the nursery I remembered the last time I sat in there, sunning my belly as Reid rolled around inside it. When for the first time after he died I felt gas bubbles move around my abdomen I burst into tears, remembering his kicks. When I stroked my necklace with the tiny bean, I remembered buying it right after finding out I was pregnant, thought of the time it was briefly lost in a sea of robes in the laundry room of a spa. A glance in the mirror at my linea nigra had me standing there, stroking it, and remembering. I felt him *there*, and *there*, and *there,* and *there*. But it was all my perception of him, never him as someone separate from me. In many ways I was grieving the loss of a part of myself as much as I was grieving the loss of someone who was once a part of me.

● ☾ ●

I'VE ONLY EVER been to one cemetery, Ohlsdorf in Germany. I was in Hamburg for modeling, and one day I had a casting scheduled near the grounds. My guidebook told me it was the biggest rural cemetery in the world, so I decided to visit. Death felt so far away from me at eighteen, and I wasn't bothered by the idea of being surrounded by it. I remember feeling surprised by how peaceful it was there. Birds flew by, their songs filtered through the branches of ancient trees that filled the grounds. Graves were marked with simple plaques, some with intricate tombstones. I read the names and dates and calculated their ages. One tombstone bore the last name Hansen, with the dates 1899–1988 underneath and a beautiful flower bed in front, a mix of magenta and white petals in bloom. I searched for a bench to sit on, then pulled out my lunch and opened up the book I was reading and took in the atmosphere.

I intended to consider this my one graveside experience. But now I'm parked in front of Vancouver's Mountain View Cemetery. I learn from a friend that there is a special dedication to infants. She said that up until the 1970s, babies that were stillborn or died shortly after birth were buried in that spot in mass unmarked graves. There was a ceremony when the memorial landscaping was finally finished in 2006 and my friend, a harpist, played the music for it. She told me that families spent time talking about their deceased child or uncle or sibling, and that for some of them it was the first time they'd been able to do so with strangers.

When I arrive, the grounds are a sea of white. In the distance, a section lined with rows of identical tombstones juts up through the snow. I look at the map I've printed and see that this is where the remains of veterans can be found. I follow the route to a large stone marking the infant area, with these words carved into its front:

> ONE STONE FOR EVERY INFANT
> Buried in this area of
> Mountain View Cemetery
> are many infants who were stillborn
> or died shortly after birth.
> One stone has been placed in this dry streambed in memory
> of each infant.
> This garden is dedicated to these little ones and their families.
> September 30, 2006

Because of the snow I can't see all of the stones, so I have no visual sense of the magnitude—though I know from what I've read that there are just shy of seven thousand in front of me. But it doesn't matter, because what I notice instead is perhaps more significant. Just ahead, there are paths of footprints carved out by recent visitors. It shows me how active the remembering is, that these are not babies that were buried decades ago and then forgotten about. I read some of the names on the stones: *John Baby Boy Oct 4–6 1963, Sarah B Miller 1936, Andrews Boy May 1940, Baby Girl Clarke Mar 2 1946*. Some of the stones have full names. Some state dates. There are large stones and small ones. When I see an exposed pile of them under a bush, around one hundred smooth surfaces glistening from the rain, I visualize the babies they are meant to represent.

I try to imagine what it must be like for these families to not know the exact spot their loved one is buried. And if spirits exist, where do those belonging to these babies go? The picture before me is a harsh one, here in the snow on frozen ground. As far as I can tell, I'm the only living person around right now.

The whole time I am here, a large crow perches at the top of the tree planted at the center of the memorial. I feel as if it is watching me, only diverting its eyes to inspect a patch of feathers beneath one of its wings. It makes me think of the novel *Grief Is the Thing with Feathers* by Max Porter, a story about a father and his two sons who are mourning the death of his wife, their mother. In it, a crow acts as a bizarre kind of grief therapist, or perhaps the crow *is* grief. In one scene the father talks to the crow about where his wife's ghost might be:

> *"If your wife is a ghost, then she is not wailing in the cup-boards and corners of this house, she is not mooching about bemoaning the loss of her motherhood or the bitter pain of watching you boys live without her."*
>
> *"No?"*

"No. Trust me, I know a bit about ghosts."

"Go on."

"She'll be way back, before you. She'll be in the golden days of her childhood. Ghosts do not haunt, they regress. Just as when you need to go to sleep you think of trees or lawns, you are taking instant symbolic refuge in a ready-made iconography of early safety and satisfaction. That exact place is where ghosts go."

Considering this now, standing atop a mass grave filled with infants, I wonder what truth this might hold for their spirits. I hope they are nowhere near this place, despite its strange beauty. But if ghosts regress, where does a baby return to? Does it remain a baby, perhaps in utero, the ultimate iconography of safety and satisfaction?

I'm glad that these children are together, though. In a situation that is overflowing with abandon, it feels right that they share this place. But I am angry that the society they were born in couldn't do more to acknowledge them. I picture the people who cared for their bodies, imagine them silently burying them in this unmarked plot, saying, "We did not see this. This does not happen." But it does happen; babies die every single day. It can't be an option to pretend otherwise.

● ☾ ●

IT IS JANUARY 4 and we have now been without Reid for more time than we were with him. This is difficult to grasp. Though no one has said it aloud, I sense that this is the end of the socially acceptable amount of time to talk about him.

Aaron and I have our final sticker to place today, and we decide to go back to the hospital, where we were nine months ago. I think back to his birth story all the time. From seeing his black head of hair fly into view after that final push to driving home in silence with an empty car seat at our backs, everything from that day will forever be sacred to us. To this day those remain the most profound moments of our lives—a time when joy and sorrow became so intertwined.

This is the first time we've driven there together since his birth. We begin at his memorial tile on one of the hospital walls. I feel vulnerable, and it all feels so painfully and beautifully familiar. The last time we were in this spot, by Admitting, it was just after midnight, and I was being wheeled to the birth suites. I remember each bump and each turn, heightened by labor. Looking at the people pass us by and the photos on the walls, you'd never guess that this place knows such intense moments of both birth and death.

When we return home, we leave his final sticker on his car seat in the nursery, and as we smooth it on we imagine what his face would have looked like squished between its straps, protesting the whole way home.

It sits patiently, waiting to be used by a future sibling, waiting to remind us of his place in our lives no matter where this journey takes us. #ninemonthswithreid has come to an end, but his presence here has not. I feel it is my responsibility to make sure it never will.

12

"PLEASE," I BEG. "Give me some hope."

I'm in my obstetrician's office, pleading with her to let me come off the birth control. My postpartum thyroiditis has now swung into the treatable hypothyroid phase, and last week my endocrinologist put me on Synthroid, a drug to provide more thyroid hormones. As soon as my new cycle started I made an appointment with the obstetrician to ask if we can start trying to conceive again.

"I'd like to see you stay on the pill another couple of months," she tells me. "We're only just starting to treat your thyroid."

I plead some more.

She hesitates, looks at something on her computer screen for a moment, and then says, "If your bleeding stops on its own, you can stay off it. But if it doesn't, or if something strange happens, I'll need you to go back on."

"Yes!" I exclaim. "Thank you."

Over the next few days my cycle continues without anything notable occurring, and with my OB's blessing, I start to take the tinctures my naturopath prescribed; I buy more ovulation tests. My body is trying to heal, and so am I.

The Synthroid is working; the dosage is right. For the first time since last summer, my thyroid hormones are finally all within the normal range. We are cleared to start our first round of fertility treatments.

Ordinarily, treatments would start after a year of trying to conceive. But given my cycle history and the fact that we were off birth control for a year and a half before conceiving Reid, our team agrees to start treatments after seven months. It doesn't matter that for much of that time my hormones and reproductive organs have been in total turmoil. I think my desperation is the deciding factor for everyone involved. Because seven months already feels like eternity.

I start taking the drug clomiphene, or Clomid, to stimulate ovulation. Immediately, I feel the side effects. Bloating, headaches, nausea. Then hot flashes. Ironically, similar to the typical symptoms of early pregnancy. I cry a lot. And scream. And throw things. I blame it on the medication and the diet (gluten-free and sugar-free and dairy-free, to help manage my thyroiditis), but that's not entirely fair. Most of my bereaved-mother friends—the ones I've made online and the local ones I connect with in person—are pregnant again. Most of them experienced losses around the same time as mine, some even months after, which shouldn't matter, but it does anyway. I am hurting. I silently pray, day and night, for their health and safety and that of their babies, but

I'm a terrible friend otherwise. I feel isolated even among the isolated.

I'm still looking for a blueprint for my future, an example of what is to come. This person had another child eleven months later, this one a year to the day, this one a year and a half. There are stories of miraculous immediate conceptions and IVF treatments and even surrogacy. Adoption is frequent too. Though I desperately hope to experience pregnancy again, I am open to any of these options. I just want to know: What will it take? When will it be my turn? Shamefully, I also want to know why others get their turn first. In my mind, we are all connected, somehow on a level playing field after losing children. So why do our futures differ so drastically? Some women will experience more losses: years of infertility, miscarriages, subsequent stillbirths, whereas others will have one, two, three healthy children without a stumble. I know that if loss doesn't favor one family over another, life after loss won't either. That's just the way things are. But I want to know. Why does God allow it? What is the plan?

I try to smile and be cheerful and congratulate these pregnant mothers, friends who have also known loss. The truth is that I *am* happy for them, and I am sad for me too. It's unfair to compare our journeys, but I can't control my feelings. I give myself permission to feel what I feel, because denying that isn't likely to help anyone.

I'm in a small exam room, hands interlaced over my abdomen, a paper-thin sheet draped across my lower half. I stare at the ceiling panels as a doctor pokes my insides with an ultrasound wand that resembles a giant dildo. I didn't ovulate on the Clomid. My family physician said that six rounds is usually all that's recommended, due to potential long-term side effects. I didn't want to waste another round, feeling that there was something wrong, something else we didn't know. So she referred me to a reproductive endocrinologist at a fertility clinic, for peace of mind. Now here I am.

"You have polycystic ovaries," the specialist, Dr. C., says suddenly. "Look," he motions to the cluster of white spots on the screen.

"What does that mean?"

"It means that this is why you're not ovulating. Your ovaries are polyfollicular—they have lots of follicles," he explains, zooming in on the spots. "See how there are over twenty, maybe even thirty?"

I squint, count them up, and nod.

"Most women have approximately five to eight. Your hormones and energy are being spent trying to grow all of these follicles. There is never one egg taking the lead, growing big enough to release."

So I was right. In a way, the diagnosis is a relief, affirming my feelings that something was off in my body.

As far as diagnoses go, we are fortunate. There are a lot of options for anovulation due to polycystic ovaries. Fertility treatments are not something we ever planned to pursue, but they are available. And I have the time. Now that we know what we're dealing with, we come up with a more specific plan. I will need different drugs, higher doses, more monitoring. "Well, it's good you were referred," Dr. C. says.

I've become that woman I swore I'd never be—the one consumed by the TTC (trying to conceive) world. The online world of acronyms like *DD* and *DS* and *BD*, of googling symptoms, avoiding alcohol, drinking decaf coffee. I have drawers full of ovulation kits and the little sticks are often sprawled out on the bathroom counter. I arrange them to look like a little fan, each leaf a reminder of what I lack. I've already shelled out more money than I want to tally up on tests and treatments: the naturopath's visits and tinctures, the visit to the doctor of Chinese medicine and their prescribed herbs, the endocrinologist's thyroid medication, the obstetrician's ovulation drugs, the ultrasound monitoring, and boxes of strips to test for ovulation and pregnancy.

I spend my days hiding under blankets and the nights I spend praying. I pray for outcomes, for results, for something positive. I see prayer used this way all around me, "prayer warriors" gathering to pray for something specific to happen. But I'm becoming less and less sure that this is the way prayer works. I still pray, though, because it's something to do. In the moments in between I lock myself in the bathroom and hold a flashlight up to the back of the pregnancy tests I've taken, examining them for a second line. Sometimes I go so cross-eyed I rip apart the tests and take out the little white strip hidden beneath the reflective glare of plastic just so I can bring it right up to my eye. Or I take a photo and upload it to a forum in the online TTC community for a "tweaker," someone who will edit the photo to reveal or disprove the existence of a positive result. They all tell me they're sorry, that there's nothing there. But maybe next month.

I wasn't prepared for how much all of this would demand of me. I heave into the toilet and wear baggy shirts to cover my bloated abdomen. I convince myself I don't care that we're doing this with medical assistance, that the pregnancy announcements that find their way to me are not meant as punishments. Though I feel desperate, I try to find solace in the fact that this is the chance at new life I've been wanting.

Why don't you just adopt? is the number-one question people ask after I open up to them about our fertility journey. It's a valid question, but I don't have a simple answer. Adoption is beautiful. There are so many children out there who need a home. It's one of the *many* beautiful ways that families can grow. But it isn't the easy way or the only way.

I know that so much healing will come from carrying another child and birthing them safely into my arms, and I'm willing to fight for that. Am I being greedy with my hopes and dreams, mistaking them for needs? Maybe. But people's reproductive decisions are so personal, and guided by reasons beyond logic.

Knowing I need to get pregnant again and knowing what I will do once I am actually pregnant again are two very different things, though. All the articles I've read on parental grief say not to get pregnant again until you no longer want the child you lost back. I still want Reid back. And I want another child. I refuse to believe those two truths can't coexist.

● ☾ ●

AARON IS AS opinionated on the treatments as he possibly can be. He doesn't like the way they transform an act he sees through the light of possibility into something that could be regarded as a failure. Like how at the end of a cycle of drugs, when the blood comes, I text him:

We're out. Can you pick up a bottle of wine on your way home?

And he doesn't want to be in a fertility clinic. Not for the way they turn something intimate into something so scientific.

"The purpose isn't for connection anymore," he says to me.

"That's not true," I assure him.

"Oh, come on," he says, irritated. "You know it is."

"What do you want me to say? That we can stop the treatments and leave things in 'God's hands'?" I use air quotations and start to shout, pacing the room, waving my arms wildly. "How fucking well did that work out for us last time?" Then I'm crying, and I try to hide it from him.

"Look." His face softens. "All I'm trying to say is the goal isn't for us to be intimate anymore, it's for me to get off so that you can get pregnant."

I will see it later, of course. Years after when I look back it will be obvious that the treatments made an ugly creature out of me. But Aaron wants another child too. And he wants one with me. So he learns to love the animal I am becoming. Or, at least, he is very good at pretending to.

Sex is a struggle; there is no pride in trying to fantasize otherwise. When we first started trying again, after Reid, I had many unresolved feelings about it. I was disconnected from my uterus, still blaming her for endangering Reid. I was reluctant about intimacy, hyperaware that he was the last to touch me there. I was frightened to open myself up again, not wanting to feel any more pain.

I did think of Reid and his birth that first time back in May, the same day I received clearance at my six-week post-partum checkup. I felt the tug of unhealed tears and the fear of what might happen. And it wasn't so bad—good, even—but it wasn't the same. Sex before death was always fun and uncomplicated for us, but like many dynamics in our new normal, this has changed too. I want to get pregnant, but the possibility also terrifies me. Sex could lead to another baby, which could lead to another loss. But I'm also terrified that it will do neither, that I will be stuck where I am. My body and mind have defaulted to that terror paradox after their trauma, a response I can't dismiss no matter how hard I try.

So we have sex, and it is clinical, stripped of emotion. It is scheduled by my doctors and my acupuncturist and discussed often by them. They grill me on things like climaxes and positions and cervical discharge. After we tell our families we are trying again, they discuss it too, though in less detail. I was never particularly shy to talk about sex before, yet this new lack of privacy suddenly makes me desperate for it.

It seems important to talk about sex after loss, though, especially since it's a topic that's rarely publicly examined. Jessica Zucker, a psychologist and the creator of the #IHadaMiscarriage campaign, wrote an essay for *New York* magazine's *The Cut* website on how her miscarriage at sixteen weeks affected her sex life. So much of her experience with intimacy after loss mirrored my own—in the terrors and dualities of it—and reading her words took away the embarrassment that existed when I thought I was alone in my feelings. She also talked about what she learned from her clients, saying:

Pregnancy loss is often associated with feelings of body betray-al—a foreboding sense that the body has "failed" or isn't doing something it's supposed to do. One common side effect is for women to retreat from sex. As a psychologist who specializes in women's reproductive and maternal mental health, I saw this for years before experiencing it myself.

Women who'd gone through miscarriage came to me express-ing how sex was the last thing they wanted, how feeling like their bodies didn't work erased the desire for intimacy. Some were afraid sex might lead to another loss, or felt guilty about not being intimate with their partners. Each time, I'd encourage them to trust their body, and their schedule. If you don't want to have sex, I told them, don't.

But we still do. Mostly, more than we want. We treat sex like a job. It is work to move through our grief to a place of intimacy, so we leave emotion out of it. I'm not sure we have any to spare.

Life feels difficult, though in the grand scheme of things, we're okay. People lose babies, or struggle to have them, all the time, and many don't have access to the support we have now. And our issue isn't that we can't ever conceive a living child (not yet); it's that we can't conceive one fast enough for our broken hearts.

I borrow Alice Jolly's acronym from her memoir *Dead Babies and Seaside Towns*, and apply it here: NRTIHRN. Noth-ing Really Terrible Is Happening Right Now. The terrible thing has happened, and this is not it. None of this is exactly ideal, but nothing really terrible is happening right now.

I know all of this. So why do I still feel so bad?

13

EASTER WILL COME before Reid's first birthday this year. Two separate anniversaries for the same monumental events of his death and birth, their dates fast approaching. I keep reminding myself: *I am here. I am okay.*

One morning, I find a little box hidden in the space above our fridge. Inside, the sole remaining cupcake from the evening we revealed Reid's sex to our family. I'm only slightly disturbed that it is still in pristine condition. I have no idea why or how we kept it, but how can I ever get rid of it now?

I think back to that anatomy ultrasound, how giddy we were with excitement, anxious for another glimpse at the human we were growing. But I have almost forgotten another detail. Halfway through the scan, a cyst was discovered on his brain. The technician, and later our doctor, explained that this was not a concern, and was only a risk if accompanied by other markers. They wouldn't even tell me what it was called because they knew I would spend the remainder of my pregnancy consulting Dr. Google. It didn't matter; the first link from my search told me it was a choroid plexus cyst, and my midwife confirmed it later when I asked. A small, fluid-filled bubble that develops on the brain of 1 to 2 percent of healthy babies. In rare cases, it can be a marker of trisomy 18, but then other abnormalities would be present.

I thought about it a handful of times over the months, but never really worried because I thought, as always: *not us*. These were the things other families had to worry about: sick babies and a lifetime of adjusting to the erasure of that "normal" child-filled future.

Now I wonder if I could have changed his fate. What if I had simply requested another ultrasound after we learned about his cyst? Aaron and I talked about it but ultimately decided to trust the doctors and limit the ultrasounds. Now I think, had we done just one thing differently, might they have discovered the knot? If we'd asked them to scan the cord, could they have seen it? Was there any possible scenario that could have led to his upcoming birthday marking a year of watching him grow instead of a year of grieving his death?

I wonder too, if the technology to detect a cord knot had been invented, and was routinely used, how would it have changed our outcome? You can't untie the knot, can you? Would I have been put on bed rest? Would I have been hooked up to machines in the hospital for months? If the knot did start to tighten, would a cesarean have saved his life? Who would make the call to let the knot tighten just a little longer rather than delivering at, say, twenty-four weeks? Would a surgery be available one day to enter the womb and pry the knot loose? And then, and then, and then. What about the countless babies that are born with true knots, healthy and very much alive?

At what cost could Reid's life have been saved? And would there ever be a price too high? What do we test and screen and intervene for? It seems impossible for me to even be thinking these things, because I want to say I would have done anything to save his life. And I would have. But at the same time, who am I to change the course of a life? More questions. So few answers.

As I prepare for Friday I wonder why they had to call it *good*—it is the most terrible holiday in our personal calendar.

I'm spending much of the week leading up hunkered down in our apartment, answering emails and writing down thoughts and watching Netflix—pressing *yes* more times than I care to admit when it prompts "Are you still watching?" It is the safest place for me now, home. I had an encounter in our building elevator earlier this week. A woman I hadn't seen since early last year was riding up with me. She commented on the weather and casually asked about "the baby," having remembered she'd last seen me heavily pregnant.

I tried to break the news gently, but she didn't take it well. She tried to recover the mood and asked if we were celebrating Easter this weekend. Poor woman, she had no idea. We both exited to our floors in tears—grief can be so unfair sometimes.

But grief can be comforting too, tender almost. There are moments when it's so sweet to be reminded of our final days with Reid. The cherry blossoms in full bloom, the scent of Ivory Snow on a stranger, the one-year-old boy with jet-black hair. The longer I live this life after loss the more I understand those mothers who told me right at the beginning that I'd never get over it, and that one day I'd be thankful for this. It's true that I've grown and changed, but my grief is still here— different, but perhaps stronger, even. I will never be the same. I don't think I should be.

We spend Good Friday on the couch, not moving for much other than to answer the door to accept a delivery of Thai food. The blinds remain drawn and we sit in the dark binge-watching *House of Cards*. We don't talk, but we don't need to. It is enough just to make it through the day, and when we do, I feel relieved. We come out the other side of the first tough anniversary, together.

I've heard so many stories of couples who are destroyed by grief, because not everyone grieves the same way. I look up the statistic and read that 80 percent of married couples who lose a child will divorce. It seems so much higher than I imagined, alarmingly so. Then I read another statistic saying the first statistic is wrong, that the prognosis is not so grim. I'm not sure what to believe, but I'm grateful that Aaron and I continue to work through life missing Reid together, even as the specifics of how we grieve often contrast. I want to talk about everything all the time, whereas Aaron, who is naturally so singularly focused, needs to set aside specific times—anniversaries, for example. We work together now, though, agreeing that we will spend this holiday at home in solitude, leaving the festive celebrations to the rest of our families. Though I have chip crumbs stuck to my sweatpants and haven't brushed my teeth, Aaron holds me close, our restless minds staving off sleep.

How did the two of us get here? I think of what Elizabeth Alexander says in her memoir *The Light of the World* about the tragic death of her husband. She writes, "The story seems to begin with catastrophe but in fact began earlier and is not a tragedy but rather a love story. Perhaps tragedies are only tragedies in the presence of love, which confers meaning to loss. Loss is not felt in the absence of love."

So does all of this begin when Aaron and I first met? I think back to that day, when it was warm and the salt from the ocean was thick in the air. My sunburnt shoulders had just started to peel. My beach volleyball partner and I were busy setting up the courts; the sun dazzled against the surface of the water north of us—a sea of diamonds, little rays of light that hit the whitecaps as the waves reached the shore.

Out of the corner of my eye, I spotted a boy I'd never seen before, walking across the parking lot. He wore impossibly short shorts in a vibrant shade of blue and a frayed straw cowboy hat—like the ones you get for free with a case of beer. Actually, I'm fairly certain it said *Budweiser* on it. A curious smile planted itself on my face as I watched this very tall, very tanned stranger wander toward us. When he took his hat off his hair, which was bleached from the sun, stood straight up. He ran his hands over it to tame it in a way that suggested he already knew it was a lost battle. "Hi, I'm Aaron," he said, still running a hand over his head.

I think of everything that followed that encounter, of the decisions we made and the motives behind them, and wonder: Why did this happen to me? Why did our child die? We are good people and somehow, over the years, I arrived at the worldview that bad things don't afflict people who are inherently good. But even before Reid's death, I must have known on some level that I couldn't be right, because I'd seen cases where good people *were* struck by the unimaginable.

Then I phrase the question differently, and it's one I *can* answer: If something this awful were to happen to anyone, why not me? The CDC states that specific groups based on ethnicity, age, specific health conditions, and financial status (to list a few) are, statistically speaking, more likely to experience stillbirth.[19] These are mostly unmodifiable factors that not only increase the risk of stillbirth but also place people at a disadvantage for support even before tragedy hits. I don't fit into these groups, so I am already at an advantage because of factors out of my control. But I can acknowledge that because of them, I *can* control what comes next. Though it should have been better, it could have been much worse. I want to find a way to use my privilege for good. I don't think I can be anyone's savior, but I might be able to accept that there's hope for something positive.

We wake up the next morning feeling lighter. In actuality, Good Friday was almost welcome—an opportunity to indulge our grief and linger in the memories. I'm learning that the lead-up to these milestone days is so agonizing that the day itself ends up being a bit of a relief. It's just a day, after all. The awful thing it commemorates has already happened. What these anniversaries really mark is a divide between the "before" and the "after"—they are another reminder that our lives have forever been split in two.

When I wake up on Reid's birthday, I want something to look forward to. I look to what other families have done on the birthdays of their babies who have passed: fundraisers, acts of kindness, book launches, charity unveilings. They are all inspiring, but I don't have the energy for them. The one thing I'm sure about is that I want this day to be about heart-centered transactions.

I think of the writing I've done, all that I've shared because of Reid and his life and his death, all who have shared in return. I think of how I am not the only one his legacy has touched. Of all of the words he has inspired in me, of all that others tell me they have learned about themselves and their own grief from reading these words.

Reid has shown me that in the year of deepest grief there is still room for big belly laughs and soft, loving moments. He has taught me how to love with both ferocity and tenderness, how to live in the present. He has motivated me to never give up. Both the importance of his brief life and the suddenness of his death have sparked something in me, something that manifests through words.

So for his birthday, we decide we will each choose one word relating to something that Reid has inspired. The easy part is coming up with a name for this celebration: Reid's Reads. I ask my blog readers to join us by choosing one word and describing what it means to them, and dedicating their thought or memory or revelation to the legacy of our son. I invite them to share this word with the world through social media. I tell them: write it down, send it out, *believe it*.

● ☾ ●

THEN, SUDDENLY, THE one-year mark is upon us. April 3 brings painful memories, and it is as if my body is remembering too. A trickling of tears and blood, an ache in my head and abdomen. I relive the day as it happened; remember in detail the hour that was the worst of my life, the ultrasounds, the Cervidil, the return home, the start of labor. We are delirious and exhausted by nightfall. Aaron and I collapse on the couch, unable to make it to bed.

In the early hours of April 4, I draft my post for Reid's birthday. I choose the word *veracity*, and as I connect it to my thoughts I describe his birth—the greatest and worst day of my life. I talk about all the things he has altered for me— beliefs and incentives. I write through two cups of coffee and an abandoned breakfast and as I do I realize that what I'm writing is a letter to Reid.

When Aaron hands me what he's written, I notice that he's framed his thoughts as a letter to Reid, too. I read his word: *presence*. He hasn't written or shared much over the year, choosing instead to work things through in his mind in silence, but hearing him reflect on the what-ifs and the impermanence of life and Reid's place in our present day reveals to me that we are working through the same things. We share a son; we share a grief. Though how we navigate these facts may differ, it is also more similar than I first noticed. It's as if by writing these letters, we are saying the same thing: that even though Reid's death means he can't receive them, he is still part of our family.

We publish our letters online, and as we get ready for the day the messages start flooding in for Reid's Reads. Eventually, there will be hundreds of them—hundreds more than I ever could have dared to hope for. I go through every single one. Some linger before me as I read and reread them, until their words find permanent residence in my mind:

> My word is saudade, *often described as "the love that remains" or "the love that stays" after someone is gone...*
> My word is share, *because sharing brings in the support needed to get through the rough parts...*
> My word is truth, *because I now know the truth; people can't hide the facts that stillbirths, miscarriages, infertility, etc. happen...*
> My word is faith. *I have been turning more toward my faith when I think of Reid, his family, and my own family that is no longer of this world.*

I collect each word, write them down: *hope, family, strength, awaken, transcendent, faith, grace, beloved, proud, grow, trust, heal, thankful, honor, skill, love, faithfulness, joy, brave, dreams, resilience, savor, grateful, home, inspire, enough, surrender, community, child, courage, fearless, longing, vulnerable, sagacity, breathe, anchor, forever, promise . . .* The list continues. I love them all.

We spend his birthday learning about all of the ways that Reid's story has touched those in our community and those well beyond it. We dared to believe this day could be met with more celebration than sorrow. And though none of these shared words have the power to change what happened, or ease the pain of moving forward without him, they do alter the way our grief lives inside us. They teach us how Reid is real for others too, and in this moment, little else is more important to us. He is thought of and talked about and incorporated into the stories of all these people.

He hasn't slipped away into nothingness.

14

P AST THE ONE-YEAR mark, I sense a noticeable shift. I'm
at a loss as to how to feel, no longer freshly grieving.
But all of a sudden, this is just how life is, and loss is
a part of my story. Things aren't easier, but the acute grief
has softened. There are days where I feel lighter. Like I can
breathe again. Like I am finally starting to break free from
the cycle of anniversaries, merging all three parallels into one.
I do not count by Fridays and Saturdays anymore, nor do I
make special note of the third and fourth of each month. For
the most part, they are just ordinary days.

A week after Reid's birthday, I have a phone meeting with
a producer who wants to include me in a reality TV show, of
all things. I ultimately decline, because the idea that my life
could provide any sort of entertainment right now is baffling,
but one part of our conversation leaves me the most confused.
The producer only recently learned of my story and mistak-
enly thought that Reid had died this year. When I correct him,

saying Reid had, in fact, died last April, he lets out a relieved, "Oh! Okay!" as if everything is fine. Was there actually a time limit on my mourning before I was ushered to move on? I hadn't realized just how many people are stuck on the old adage, "Time heals all wounds." I don't believe that to be the least bit true. Yes, some healing has occurred. The debilitating pain has subsided and memories of the trauma have softened a bit around the corners. The wound is still there, though; it just looks different now. Not quite a scar yet, but no longer gaping, raw, and exposed. It will always be present in some form, I imagine.

Amid the confusing period of transitioning beyond the first year, I am starting to feel a little more human, a little more familiar. And I am still searching to know who it is that I'm growing to become.

I have done a lot since last April, but I have also done very little. A lot of days spent indoors, reading books, writing stories and posts, connecting with bereaved parents online, watching bad television. I am working part-time as a model and teach a weekly yoga class, but on the recommendation of my doctor I have had to stop attending the births that would complete my doula training. Assisting these births was disrupting my cycle and causing more bleeding, complicating fertility treatments, and my doctor told me I had to make a choice.

The choice is simple: we want another baby. We take a look at our budget and decide that I can put the doula dream aside and be selective with work. I eliminate stressors where possible, seek social safety when I can, tuck myself away from as many human interactions as possible. In this post-loss world, social situations have become exhausting. I have always been an introvert, though perhaps more of an extroverted one—loving a good gathering of people but recharging best with my own company. But grief has made me a true recluse. And after the first year this is still as true as ever. Even something as mundane as making small talk with the barista at a café weighs me down. We can talk about the weather, work, plans for the rest of the day. I'll be on autopilot and reply with short and courteous answers, but I'll just be thinking about Reid. I'm always thinking about Reid, or keeping him close to my thoughts. And I wish I could talk about him too. But saying "Oh, my plans? I should be going for a stroll at the beach with my son, but he was stillborn last year" to the barista isn't exactly what I want to be doing either.

Time keeps going by; treatments progress and are altered as they fail. Because I'm still not ovulating, we are starting to put IVF on our radar, budgeting accordingly. In the meantime, drug dosages are upped, ultrasounds continue, appointments are scheduled. More visits and treatments and testing and waiting.

It's easy to say "Just one more month" when the fertility clinic asks if we want to continue. Nothing outside of motherhood matters to me anymore, and I am only marginally aware of how small my life has become. It has shrunk right down to this obsessive world of monitoring my fertility and trying to conceive. I have no emotional or mental capacity to entertain anything else. How have we gotten here?

Clomid is swapped for another drug, Letrozole, also known as Femara. This drug is commonly used as a cancer-fighting medication, and this is already enough to make me nervous. Then Dr. C., my reproductive endocrinologist, tells me that if I google it I will find coverage of a study linking it to an increase in birth defects. He says not to worry, that the correlation has since been disproven. He hands me a piece of paper detailing all of this and I read it daily.

When we are on our third medicated cycle, the second on the Letrozole, I receive a call from our fertility clinic while shooting on set. "I'm so sorry," the nurse begins, "but you didn't ovulate this time either."

I press my index finger and thumb into the bridge of my nose and let out a sigh. The makeup artist gives me a look. I mouth a silent apology for smudging the makeup and hold up my finger to tell her I'll just be a minute. "Okay," I say to the nurse. "What do we do now?"

I hear the clicking of a mouse and the whir of a distant printer in the background as she books me in to see Dr. C. later that day to investigate what has happened.

"I'm not sure why you didn't ovulate," Dr. C. tells me at our ultrasound in the afternoon. "But your lining looks good, so I think we'll skip your next period and give you the same high dose of Letrozole to start taking tonight." It seemed that perfectly good-looking sixteen-millimeter follicle that had shown on our ultrasound a week earlier had just vanished, regressed when it should have released.

"Is that safe to take the drugs again so soon?" I ask.

"Absolutely," he answers. "It's no different than starting treatments on any other cycle."

He books me in for another scan in nine days. If we see a follicle over seventeen millimeters, this time I will take an injection of human chorionic gonadotropin—hCG—to force the egg to release.

The next morning I wake up to blood. I call Dr. C.; he tells me the bleeding should stop soon, that I should keep taking the drugs. I'm doubtful, remembering the last time I heard similar words and I bled for forty-one days. But Dr. C. tells me that he hasn't given up. And there's the hope again, the thing that appears whether I want it or not, the feeling that keeps me going.

Today is Friday: ultrasound day. I show up at the clinic with very low expectations. So when Dr. C. and I are left staring at a screen that shows two large follicles, at seventeen and twenty millimeters, we are speechless.

After the scan I spend a few minutes with my favorite nurse learning how to administer the hCG injection. She is entertained by me, I think. Laughing as I take photos and notes of everything she shows me.

"The actual needle won't hurt," she assures me. "Just remember: quick for the jab into the skin and slow for the release of the medication."

"Show me again?" I ask. I pull out my phone and take a video, laughing with her as I shake my head in disbelief that this is where I've ended up.

After I'm done, we hug goodbye and she whispers, "Good luck!" I thank her, hold up crossed fingers, and she does the same before waving excitedly as I walk out the door.

I leave the clinic with a tiny hundred-dollar syringe filled with human chorionic gonadotropin; my wallet is a little lighter, but my spirits are too. We have a plan, and for the first time in a long time, I have faith in it.

The next day is injection day. We've been told to do it at two in the afternoon. Aaron and I drive out to visit his family an hour out of the city, the shot in a cooler in the back seat. We arrive shortly after one o'clock. I take the syringe out and let it sit at room temperature, as instructed, then pace Aaron's parents' home as I watch the time pass on the digital screen below the stove.

Aaron is sweating. I'm too nervous to do the shot myself so he will give it to me, but he's starting to look a little pale. I see him practice a stabbing motion, then shake his head. By two o'clock, he is absolutely adamant that he will not be the one to inject me. Derek's fiancée, Angela, a nurse, is also there, and she graciously volunteers.

It's a family event, quite literally. Months ago, Aaron and I discussed in great detail whether to include our whole family in this process of trying to conceive, but we ultimately decided it wasn't something we needed to keep secret. They are our biggest supporters, after all, and this is the most important thing happening in our lives right now. It also feels important for them to know that we're doing something that gives us hope. We're trying to make a baby. That's something to celebrate.

It's a unique feeling when the people closest to you have intimate knowledge of your cycle and conceiving efforts. I lean back in the wide leather chair and Hank, Annette, Derek, Levi and his girlfriend (Katie), Hanah, Carson, and Aaron gather around as Angela cleans an inch of skin next to my belly button. A quick pinch of fat and a stab and it is all over. I feel the uncomfortable sensation of the medication spreading through my body. Within a few hours, the effects have subsided to a little bloating, mild nausea, and a headache. It's manageable. It's working.

Our next few days look a little something like this:

"It's sex day," I say. "When do you want to do it?"

"Now's good?" Aaron asks.

"Okay," I reply, before I realize that I need to shower.

"I could use one too," Aaron says, then winks as he adds, "We could shower together?"

I think of all the reasons I should say yes. It would be fun and spontaneous, which we could use right now. But then I think about what I need more, that obsessive desire to conceive taking over. "We should probably do it in the bed," I answer. "That way I can put my legs up against the wall right after."

"Ah yes," Aaron states. "Okay, sounds good."

Around this time I read *When Breath Becomes Air* by Paul Kalanithi. I am enthralled by the words this man wrote, knowing his own end was fast approaching, about his search for what made life meaningful. But it is his unique perspective as a medical professional—a neurosurgeon—that most fascinates me. When faced with a cancer diagnosis with the statistics against him, he examined the role of hope as he and his wife, Lucy, went to a fertility clinic to freeze "gametes and options":

> *The word* hope *first appeared in English about a thousand years ago, denoting some combination of confidence and desire. But what I desired—life—was not what I was confident about—death. When I talked about hope, then, did I really mean "Leave some room for unfounded desire"? No. Medical statistics not*

only describe numbers such as mean survival, they measure our confidence in our numbers, with tools like confidence levels, confidence intervals, and confidence bounds. So did I mean "Leave some room for a statistically improbable but still plausible outcome—a survival just above the measured 95 percent confidence interval"? Is that what hope was? Could we divide the curve into existential sections, from "defeated" to "pessimistic" to "realistic" to "hopeful" to "delusional"? Weren't the numbers just the numbers? Had we all just given in to the "hope" that every patient was above average?

It occurred to me that my relationship with statistics changed as soon as I became one.

I spend time on the Sunday that I read those words making art out of my breakfast, sipping hot coffee, and rereading them over and over. Though Kalanithi's experience with death was different from mine, his words resonate. Could he have hoped for survival? And with it, for the chance to see the children he desired to conceive grow?

Hope has seeped in and out of my heart often during the past year; it comes and goes as it pleases. As a woman rooted in science who stumbled into faith as an adult, I feel this paragraph explains so exactly what I am wrestling with. Does the science back my hope? And if so, does it really matter? I was the "above average" patient in my pregnancy, and death still found us. Someone has to be the one in a thousand. And yet, hope is crucial to life. Without hope—hope for change, hope for salvation, hope for a good life for ourselves and our neighbors—what are we doing here?

So I hope for a different outcome than the one my history arrived at: that if we have another baby, this hope is reasonable. For, as Kalanithi also wrote, "Science may provide the most useful way to organize empirical, reproducible data, but its power to do so is predicated on its inability to grasp the most central aspects of human life: hope, fear, love, hate, beauty, envy, honor, weakness, striving, suffering, virtue."

But aren't we all just hoping against the odds? The one statistic we can be completely sure of is that 100 percent of us will die. At some point in our lives, we will all experience devastating loss. So what are we really hoping for?

"I have your results," the nurse that coached me through the injection says over the phone.

I breathe deeply.

"Are you ready?" she asks.

"Tell me," I reply.

"You ovulated!" she exclaims.

Ah yes, I think. *This. This is what we were hoping for.* For the first time since I became pregnant nearly two years earlier I finally have a chance to get pregnant again.

Then she adds, "And your progesterone levels are so high that we think both of your follicles released eggs. So there's a possibility of twins if you do conceive this time!"

The nurse schedules my pregnancy test for next Friday, the full moon, and I take this coincidence as a good omen. She tells me that I can take a home pregnancy test starting this Sunday, if I really need to, and reminds me that it will be positive at first because of the hCG trigger: I can test to see the hormone leave my system, and then test again for pregnancy after.

She must know that testing early and often is a frequent thing while trying to conceive, because this is exactly what I will do.

I tell Aaron the news, pass it on to eagerly awaiting family. Everyone is notably relieved. They are excited that I have ovulated, and nervous about the happiness they hear in my voice. I keep reassuring them that no matter what happens we will be fine because at least we have real hope now; at least we know my body can ovulate again.

The week drags on, and when it has finally been seven days I pull out one of the Clearblues I have on hand, knowing I'll get a false positive. The last time I saw two pink lines on a First Response test was when I found out I was pregnant with Reid, and I don't want to see them again until I'm ready to actually test for pregnancy. I watch the faint little blue cross appear, then note it down and throw the test out.

On Monday, I take another test, and this time the second line is barely visible. Then on Tuesday, ten days after my injection, my test is completely negative. Any positives going forward will be the real deal.

I think of how intentional we are being with the conception of this future child. I think of how it was with Reid. He was unplanned. Wanted, and also a surprise. I want to forget that little detail of his story that seems so insignificant, but I can't. I pick every aspect of it apart. This truth doesn't give me any less permission to grieve him, does it?

Once Levi asked Aaron and me what we would tell Reid about his unexpected appearance in our lives. We were sitting in the living room as Annette and Hanah made dinner.

"I mean," he started to say. "*I* was an accident."

"Oh, Levi!" Annette shouted at him as she checked the slow cooker.

"What?" he exclaimed. "Just look at the age gap between Hanah and me compared to her and Derek or Aaron. You could have fit at least one more child in there."

Annette laughed. "You were not an accident."

"We'll probably be honest and tell him he was a surprise," I said lightly.

"Really?" Hanah asked.

"It doesn't change how much we love him now," Aaron replied. Then he added, "Or how much we have always wanted him."

"Exactly," I said. "The best surprise." And I believed it, because I also still believed that the best things were often unexpected.

At seven thirty on Wednesday morning, I take a First Response test. And for the first time since I found out I was pregnant with Reid, there is a second pink line. Granted, it is a very, very faint one, but I don't need flashlights or sunlight to see it. It is there, and I can't believe that, a year after first wishing it into existence, another baby might be too.

I don't dare jinx or curse or assume by saying that I definitely, without a doubt am pregnant. I can't let myself go there. But I have to tell Aaron. I walk slowly back into the bedroom and, fighting back tears, with that pregnancy test clutched tightly in my hand, whisper that I can see a tiny second line. He is half asleep, squinting to see what I'm showing him. I'm not sure he believes me. But I recognize a glimmer of happiness in his eyes that I haven't seen in a very long time.

That night I hardly sleep a wink. It reminds me of the anticipation I always felt on Christmas Eve as a child, knowing I'd wake up to sticky pastries and carols and gift giving in the morning. Six-thirty rolls around and I can't wait a minute longer. I hop out of bed and take the next test. I set my timer and pour myself a glass of icy cold water from the fridge. When the harp of my alarm starts to strum I walk back to the bathroom and hover over the test. Two pink lines, the second one darker than the test from yesterday.

I run into our room and jump on Aaron until he wakes up. Begrudgingly, he blinks his eyes open and musters enough energy to hit me with a pillow and mumble, "Why are you awake?!"

I hand him the test and smile. "The second line is darker today. I think this is really it. I think I'm actually pregnant!" I think back to the false positive I got in New York once, think of second lines that don't get darker with a chemical pregnancy, think about very early miscarriage. This isn't any of those right now, I'm sure of it.

Aaron sees it this time, that second pink line, stares at it a little longer to make sure. He gives me a big squeeze and a bunch of little kisses and pulls me back down, tries to convince me to get a little more sleep. But I escape his grasp. I can't lie still. Everything is changing, going a million miles a minute. I have this peculiar awareness of needing to catch up.

On the morning of the full moon I wake up early and take another test to brace myself for whatever news might come our way from the blood test scheduled today. Two pink lines, the second even darker still. With that knowledge I walk down to the lab, the same one where I'd done my first pregnancy blood test with Reid. In the room, the woman taking my blood smiles.

"Do you know the answer to this test?" she asks.

"This is the first blood test," I say. "So I don't know anything for sure."

She nods and wishes me luck as she sticks a bandage on my arm, and I leave with my phone already open to the online results. I spend the rest of the day refreshing my account every ten minutes on my computer, then on my phone when I have to leave the apartment. I'm really not a patient person.

Aaron and I want to make our announcement to family special if there is good news; this maybe-baby deserves the same as Reid. We figure if the blood test is negative, we'll want to be around family anyway, and if it confirms what we already suspect then we'll have everyone together to share in our joy. We ask our parents to gather the siblings and grandparents and meet us for dinner at an outdoor restaurant, not telling them both sides of the family are invited. Wondrously, they don't suspect a thing.

I get messages all day:

Do you know anything yet?

Are you okay?

Anything?

Hello?

???

I ignore them all, and after each text I refresh my online account. I feel I will surely lose my mind in the waiting, and yet, I'm equally sure that the news will be good.

When it's time to leave for dinner the results still aren't in. I have no idea what we'll do if we don't find out before having to face our families. The drive to the restaurant is thirty minutes from our apartment and I keep hitting *refresh* every two minutes, then every thirty seconds. Just as we are about to leave the city limits they appear. Before I click to open them I see a tiny pink *Y* signifying "Results out of range" and remember that is something you want when hoping for pregnancy. I look to Aaron and whisper, "They're in." I hold my breath and open the file and there are my hCG levels:

42 IU/L

In the third week of pregnancy they should be between 5 and 50.

"It's positive!" I squeal, dropping the phone to squeeze Aaron's thigh.

He beams at me. "You're pregnant?!" He grabs my hand and pulls it up to give it a kiss.

"I'm pregnant! I'm really pregnant!" Right there in our trusty old Ford Focus, driving down Granville Street with the glow of the full moon shining hazily through the rain clouds, we find out that our family of three is finally a family of four. Then I recall what the nurse said about releasing two eggs. "Gosh, what if it's twins?" we wonder aloud, and it feels familiar. All of it. And it is impossible not to think of Reid. We feel his presence so strongly, receiving this news on the full moon of his birth month. The start of our emergence from a year of very deep grief.

Maybe what I needed all along was to get through a whole year of grieving and loving Reid exclusively before my body could make room for new life. The happiness I feel in that car, the kind that always seems to flutter just beyond my reach, spreads its wings and turns and soars right toward me. I embrace it and stroke its wings and laugh at its return. I've missed it. I've missed it dearly.

In the parking lot of the restaurant, just as the rain starts to fall, both sides of our family arrive at the same time. As they walk closer to us, the squeals begin.

"What?" Hanah exclaims. "What are *they* doing here?" She points to my family. I hold up my phone and start to record, trying to conceal my face behind the screen as we wait for everyone to gather together before us. Rebecca starts jumping up and down, clutching the hand of her boyfriend, Trenton. Levi and Katie are grinning. Our parents embrace. Derek and Angela are watching us carefully. Alana is waving her hands expectantly; her boyfriend, Jeremy, has a hand on her shoulder. Carson crosses his arms, smiling proudly at us.

"Oh, go on," my grandmother says. "You've got your mother in tears!" She starts to weep herself.

With a quick wink, Aaron and I shout, "We're pregnant!"

Everyone screams happily. There are tears, hugs, smiles. Strangers peer at us curiously as they walk by, trying to figure out what is going on. The restaurant has closed for the evening, but we don't care. We order takeout from our favorite pizza place and take the food back to my parents' home at the end of the village. There is champagne (and sparkling lemonade), fueling animated conversations and laughter that fill the room.

As I scan the faces of all the ones we hold dear, I note that the last time I saw each of them so happy was when we were all in this same room, having a party for Reid when I was pregnant with him. They have been through everything with us, and this baby, this long-awaited baby, is theirs to celebrate too. We all linger in the room, talking, laughing, and dreaming once again. No one wants to leave and I can't blame them. The atmosphere is blissful. I would be quite happy to sit here all night long.

● ☾ ●

I DREAM OF Reid for the second and last time shortly after I find out I'm pregnant again. I know in an instant that it's him. He is with me, Aaron, and Derek, and we are coming back from a road trip, driving in a black SUV. Aaron is at the wheel and I'm in the passenger seat. Derek is in the back with Reid, who is about five or six, his long limbs seeming to protrude to impossible lengths. He's letting out really terrible-smelling farts and we are all doubled over with laughter. Each one has us plugging our noses and rolling down the windows, gasping for air as we catch the breeze with our faces.

After a few minutes of this, he looks up at me in the mirror with a stoic gaze and asks for a juice box.

"Did I hear a please?" I ask, raising my eyebrow.

"Yep," he responds smartly. Then, when he realizes I'm not budging, he lets out an exasperated sigh. "Puh-leeze?" He draws out the *e* sound and bounces his outstretched hand impatiently.

I fish one out of my backpack and place it in his sweaty little palm. It's an apple and orange combo—his favorite. He drinks silently, drawing the sweet liquid up through the straw in earnest. He makes sure to slurp every last drop and when he finishes he hands the sticky box back.

I study his face in the rearview mirror. He is handsome. His short, black hair sticks up in every direction and his skin looks tanned next to the stark white of his T-shirt. Shiny blue shorts hit his legs just above his knobby knees. He looks like I did around that age. Except his nose—that is definitely his father's nose.

I wonder if this dream could be a gift from Reid. Or is it God? How does that go? I sometimes imagine Reid sitting next to a large formless man on a pink, fluffy cloud. Reid kicking his feet around over the edge as they talk and watch us go about our lives. Reid might turn to God and say, "I think my mom could really use a dream of me right now," and He will probably nod. "Yes, good idea." I turn this scene over in my mind and decide it isn't too fanciful to believe. Just the right amount of angels and goodness.

15

WHEN I LOOK down, I see blood. It's Mother's Day, and Aaron and I were curled up together, tired from an emotionally charged day. The celebrations were joyful, the new baby bringing a kind of ease, though grief was still present. We've been watching *Game of Thrones*. The Red Wedding massacre was just on, with Robb Stark's pregnant wife stabbed repeatedly in her abdomen. I excused myself and went to the bathroom, feeling some mild cramping. I'm in the habit of checking my underwear for blood every time I go, and when I cast my eyes down, it was there. I cry out for Aaron and show him the streaks of red. We are both frozen in our thoughts. I ask him what we should do, even though I know that there's very little hope if what we think is happening is actually happening. We never say it aloud, but miscarriage seems like the most logical outcome.

I page my doctor shortly before midnight and he books us for an early ultrasound the next morning. All night I check for more bleeding. Each time I do there is a little more.

When we wake, we drive to the clinic in silence. There is silence in the elevator and the waiting room and the exam room. Neither of us knows what to say. Dr. C. starts the ultrasound and immediately checks the heart. A tiny speck flickers away at 104 bpm inside a sweet-pea-shaped blob measuring right on track for six weeks. I'm so thankful to hear the words "And there's the heartbeat!" that I don't even process the fact that we are seeing this baby for the first time.

The whole thing is bittersweet. Bitter because we ached to hear those words last April, and sweet because this baby is alive and well. Apparently some bleeding in early pregnancy can be normal, common even. While obviously it can also be a warning sign of bad news to come, it isn't always. It crosses my mind to ask if the bleeding could have been from the second egg, a possible twin. But I never do.

I know that this will only be the first of these moments. Ones where we'll fear for our second child's life and doubt that we'll ever get the chance to hold them in our arms. Our mourning has made us superstitious, and now we search for guarantees wherever we can. This doesn't help. The physical evidence isn't supporting what I'm trying to convince myself of: that this baby will make it home with us. Aaron keeps whispering in my ear, "It'll be okay." I'm not sure if he's talking about the bleeding or what will come after, but he makes me feel better. He has a way of doing that.

I am ten weeks pregnant, which means we have our first appointment with our new high-risk obstetrician, Dr. B. I first met her briefly at the International Stillbirth Alliance conference I attended back in October while on a writing assignment, where she spoke about the specific care she offered during pregnancies after late-term losses. I decided then that I would seek her out when I got pregnant again, knowing I would be considered high risk because most pregnancies after stillbirth are.

Walking into her office, I immediately feel comfortable. She has a happy lamp on her desk and wears a patterned blouse. She is a no-nonsense kind of woman but has a quirky sense of humor. On her wall is a calendar she made, with Photoshopped images of herself doubled to appear as a twin; she wears glasses, her twin does not. This is her way of celebrating her clients, as a high-risk obstetrician who deals primarily with twin pregnancies, and she has their birth dates entered in every month. She even hosts an annual doubles party, she says.

We arrive at that first appointment unprepared for the emotions it will bring up. I give a urine sample, have my blood pressure taken, get weighed. All things I did at my last prenatal appointment, just three days before Reid passed away. A whole new world of second firsts opens up now. It puts me in a dreamlike trance and fills me with more sadness than I predicted. Aaron and I sit in the waiting room and talk about how strange it feels to be back here, in the journey through pregnancy, and how different it feels too.

I'm determined not to cry. I want to seem like a level-headed person who has her grief under control and is fully prepared to be pregnant again. Dr. B. sees right through me. "I know that this must be terrifying for you. You are allowed to be scared," she says. She puts her pen down and looks at me from across the table. "But I promise you we are going to get this baby to you alive."

Heavy tears burst out of me, loud ones that I can't control. She hands me one of those tiny packs of tissues that really aren't tissues but tiny squares of thin, nonabsorbent paper. I try to blot the mess of salty water off my face anyway. I know she can't make that promise, but she sounds so confident that I decide to believe her.

"Here's my cell phone." She jots ten little numbers onto a Post-it. "You call or text me anytime. If you're going crazy and need a quick little scan, just let me know."

I clutch that piece of paper to my heart all the way home.

I'm not sure there's anything quite like being pregnant again after stillbirth. You're filled with fear and hope, and you feel these things simultaneously, though not always equally. Sometimes the fear wins and your mind goes to those deep, dark places. When you're dealing with fear based on experience, you can't tell your brain the same stories you would about other kinds of fears, that they're "not real" or "unlikely." Besides, you're back in the same physical state your loss happened in. Then sometimes the hope wins. You find yourself dreaming of stroller walks and first days of preschool and weddings before you even consider stopping yourself. And then sometimes you're somewhere in the middle, in a state similar to numbness, where you think it simply can't be real, it's not happening. You have to give yourself permission to both mourn and celebrate, to feel or acknowledge whatever it is that does or doesn't come up, and let go of any guilt you have about the emotions that emerge. You have to know that there is no single right way to do it.

I imagined myself reacting in two different ways after finding out I was pregnant again. In the first, which I suspected I'd lean toward, I would avoid celebrations and nicknames and talking about anything that might happen after the baby was born. In the second, I would do the exact opposite. I surprised myself by acting out this second scenario. We told friends and family that same day. We announced the news on all of my social media platforms and to my readers two days after that. I bought maternity clothes and baby clothes. I planned a shower.

Honestly, I want to celebrate every single moment I get with this baby. I want them to have the same experiences as their big brother.

Amelia Barnes spoke to this in her book, *Landon's Legacy*, writing about her own pregnancy after loss. She said:

> *There is nothing harder than being a parent to a child not on this earth and then opening your heart to love another child when you know there are no guarantees.*
>
> *But when you do, you realize there is really nothing that can stand in your way. When you let go of fear and stop trying to shield yourself from pain, but rather let it move in and through you, it no longer has the power to shape and control your life. You stop wasting energy on protecting your sensitive spots and seeking ways to stop bad things from happening because you realize this is a far more painful burden than feeling raw pain itself.*

A natural reaction to loss is that you start to anticipate more traumas, thinking, *the worst has already happened, why wouldn't it happen again?* Even when you're told it's unlikely, or maybe that's exactly why—the unlikely trauma has happened before, and somehow it seems more probable that it will repeat itself. So you fight like hell to prevent that thing from coming, and you try to find control where you can.

But I don't want to let fear steal any possible joys away from me now that I'm pregnant again. Even though I've never been more terrified, I don't want to let that dictate the way I live or the way I feel about this baby. I want to talk about them and dream about them. I have to do more than say no to the panic. As Amelia said, I have to find a way to accept that these life-altering events could come for me again. I can't let this possibility debilitate me. And though I understand this, though I am working to accept it, it is still a difficult truth to bear.

● ☾ ●

WE ARE GIVEN an estimated due date: January 2, 2017. However, we will induce labor at thirty-eight weeks, as is often standard practice for a pregnancy after a late-term stillbirth, usually in an effort to minimize anxiety and avoid reaching the point of pregnancy where the previous baby died. So this baby will come in mid- to late December. A Christmas baby.

Our families do not miss the significance of this. That Reid passed away at Easter and that this child is due to arrive at Christmas feels too symbolic. Part of me wants to fall to my knees and worship the God who ordained it. The other part wants to scream out against how scripted our lives seem. Are we just pawns in some big play?

I've been struggling with the faith I clung to so fiercely after Reid died. That prophetic light that Aquinas wrote of, that feeling I had during his birth and in the first weeks and months after, is gone now. Where I initially found support in religion, I now find fear. It feels like understanding death—enduring it—is in some way inviting its untimely possibility back in. And I am decidedly reluctant to put my trust in one conviction again.

I also want to believe that this connection means something. In the beginning, this search for meaning and the thought that it could exist as a reason for his death was comforting. But as the pain broke through the shock and took up residence inside of me, it shattered the comfort I'd found in the process. Because if there is a reason, do I really want to hear it?

As I soften to surrender now, I think of Ann Voskamp:

I wonder too . . . if the rent in the canvas of our life backdrop, the losses that puncture our world, our own emptiness, might actually become places to see. To see through to God. That that which tears open our souls, those holes that splatter our sight, may actually become the thin, open places to see through the mess of this place to the heart-aching beauty beyond. To Him. To the God we endlessly crave.

This gift, the promised birth of a Christmas child after the Easter death of his brother, repairs a small part of the sense of faith I crave to experience once again. It does not promise a certain outcome. It does not bend details into order. But it's as if God whispers: *See? I am here.* It feels like the support I'll need to journey through another pregnancy.

However, the significant dates are not guarantees, so I take matters into my own hands too. We decide to abstain from sex. I frequently imagine that the baby could be jostled into tying a knot. It isn't logical, but there it is. I do what's necessary to stay sane. I do what we need to survive. Love, at that most biologically intimate level, is somehow not part of that. And I have to trust that I'll know when it can be once more.

● ☾ ●

I'M CONVINCED THAT the baby is a girl. I know that sex doesn't define a child, that they could identify as someone else and we would love them no differently for it, but knowing that Reid was a boy gave me what I felt was a deeper sense of connection to him during pregnancy—it was one of the few things that we did get to learn about him. So we agree to find out through a test that can detect the baby's DNA in my blood. We are doing it to test for any trisomies that might result in stillbirth or neonatal death; the early reveal of the sex is just a bonus.

As we wait, I pick out a name, redecorate the nursery, and style her in my mind with an ease that surprises me. To imagine a little girl makes it seem less like we are inserting a new child into the life another was meant to live. I grieve the idea of what I imagined raising a son would be like, and resolve to sort out those feelings as quickly as possible.

When I'm just shy of twelve weeks pregnant, the results of the test come back: we're having another boy. Dr. B. declares it by text, followed by five enthusiastic exclamation marks, and sends me a photo of the test results to prove it. A squealing, milky little brother for Reid. I try not to think about how male babies have a higher risk of stillbirth, or how this feels a little more like a second chance instead of a separate experience altogether. I don't know what to do with Reid's things or how to go about preparing a room for another son.

I read the results again, focus on the words *low risk* beside the various fatal conditions listed. There is less than a 0.01 percent chance of any of these things resulting in an early death for this baby. Though it's not completely impossible, it's enough that I can breathe. As far as we know, he is healthy. Now we just have to hope that we continue to stay on the life-giving side of the statistics, and if we do, that it means we'll get to bring him home.

I am walking around an abandoned racetrack with my friend Tara and her one-and-a-half-year-old son, Chayton, having just finished a picnic lunch in the center of the track. I am early in my second trimester, my belly now noticeable. We pause in the shade to cool off from the penetrating heat of the afternoon summer sun. I fold down the extra fabric of my maternity jeans, scrunch up my tank, and drink the last of my water. While we chat we watch Chayton play with sticks and explore hollow tree trunks. I think back to the last time I was pregnant in his presence, heavily pregnant with Reid, attempting to soothe his newborn cries as I held him and feeling a commotion of kicking from inside me as I did. It seemed as if Reid was saying, "Hey, keep it down out there!" I told Tara and she joked, "Either that or he's objecting in solidarity with his friend."

As we stand there, a spotted orange monarch appears, makes a few quick circles around us, and promptly lands on my hand. He stays there for what must be at least five minutes before flying off to a nearby leaf. I've never had a butterfly linger on my skin before.

Then, a few seconds later, the butterfly loops back and lands on the same hand again, near my belly. He stays there for long enough that I can take some photos before he flies away, circles back, and lands on my chest. He is on me for about fifteen minutes before we finally make our way out of the woods, leaving me and Tara in complete awe.

Whatever that visit was, I can't help but feel there was a certain kind of magic to it, a comfort, maybe. Of course I don't believe the butterfly was Reid, or that he sent it. Though part of me doesn't think either is impossible, for I often feel him all around me, in the fullness of a moon or an oddly shaped reflection of light on a wall. What I do know is that I don't have to examine it. It can be nothing, or it can be a wondrous miracle—a sign that many unknowns exist in our world.

When I return home with sun-kissed skin and swollen feet, I look at my calendar and realize that it is July 12—two years to the day since we conceived Reid. As I sit there basking in the connection, I feel the first clear pokes from the baby boy growing inside of me. It feels like an undeniable, God-ordained moment of comfort. Too beautiful to be random. I prefer to leave it at that.

● ☾ ●

I AM DIAGNOSED with gestational diabetes and referred to a specialist clinic. I can tell that the doctor has been doing this for a long time, and has been hardened by the years of telling pregnant people they can't indulge in their cravings for sugar or ice cream or carbs.

At my first appointment, I am given a testing kit that fits into a little black zip-up case. I sit around a table with another pregnant patient, both of us new to this. There is a schedule: test seven times a day, one day off, then four times, another day off, then four times, third day off, test two times, repeat. First thing, before bed. An hour before meals, an hour after, sometimes both. A nurse is across from us, telling us that it is very important that we follow every instruction carefully.

"Your baby could *die* if you don't," she says.

I stare at her, wonder if I should tell her that I know this. I know.

We are driving to visit Hank and Annette at their acreage in the suburbs. The city views give way to rolling landscapes. "Do you ever wonder—" Aaron starts, then pauses, glancing at me thoughtfully from the driver's seat. "If in some way this might be Reid coming back again? I mean, how do we know?"

"No," I answer so harshly that I practically spit. I feel him recoil from me.

"I know. I know it's not. But I do wonder." He is visibly hurt and I immediately regret lashing out, surprised by how closed off I am to the idea. I, who notices glimpses of our firstborn all around me, can't even tolerate the thought that it might be possible?

I pause, take a breath, ask him to tell me more about what he is thinking. He talks to me of other cultures that abide by this—that spirits can be born again. It's a belief in many Eastern religions—Jainism, Hinduism, Buddhism, Sikhism. So, he asks, why can't we press into that? With the options on offer—that spirits enter an eternal heaven or hell, that they go nowhere and die with the body, that they enter their own spirit world, that they linger among us, or that they are born again—is rebirth somehow less logical than any of the others?

Hearing this, I don't think Aaron's unreasonable for wanting to talk about the possibility of bonding with his firstborn son the way he always imagined. I'm glad we're able to talk about these things. Because the truth is, I want it too. I would do anything for another chance to parent Reid, wouldn't I? I have asked that same question, just in a different way. But it suddenly seems a slippery slope, an unfair belief to impose on this new being. Won't it already be heavy enough to enter a home where an unfulfilled life exists? He won't need his parents' burdening belief that he is someone else. Not before he even has the opportunity to learn who he is for himself.

Aaron rarely says anything during our doctor's appointments. He sits in the chair reserved for partners and clutches the armrests, holding his breath. He's distant and quiet, entirely unlike himself, and Dr. B., noticing, always tries to make him laugh. When he doesn't, I try to make up for it and laugh twice as loudly as I normally would, looking nervously between the two of them.

"Hey," I say after an appointment one day, thinking carefully about how to ask him about this. "Do you like Dr. B.?"

"What?" he replies. "Yeah, she's great. Why do you ask?"

"It's just, you don't laugh at her jokes. She tries so hard to get you to smile," I explain.

"Don't I?" he says, surprised. "I think she's funny, really I do. I'm just always bracing myself for bad news."

I hadn't considered that up until the time for the ultrasound, he sat there feeling as helpless as he had when we were told that Reid was dead. He couldn't feel that the baby was kicking as we talked. How difficult it must feel to relinquish so much control in this situation. His importance in that room is undeniable, but he must feel like a bystander.

We mention this at the next appointment, and I stop trying to laugh for him. A new dynamic is established and his anxiety is acknowledged alongside mine. Dr. B. and I continue to banter about this or that and Aaron sits holding those armrests, but I make sure to talk about how much the baby is moving, how I feel his hiccups, how his feet press into my ribs. His grip loosens a little as I do. Aaron lost a child too, and he is going through pregnancy again with me. This journey is our burden and our joy to share.

Things Aaron does to help keep me sane:

- Rearranges furniture. A bed through one doorway into another room and then back again, slightly to the side, then closer to the window. All because it didn't *feel* right.

- Listens to me vent my anxiety about not feeling movement, and understands when I explain that once I can
  feel it, I am still anxious, but for different reasons.
- Helps me remember the things I can't: where I put my
  keys (usually the fridge), or when to brush my teeth.
- After my gestational diabetes diagnosis, keeps sugar out
  of the house and gives up chips. Chips! This is huge.
- Bonds with this baby, giving him his own nickname
  and talking to him.
- Builds shelves from scratch for the nursery when the
  ones I find and *just need to have* are $800.
- Lets me know when I need a reality check. Like when
  I learn about a certain thing so-and-so's doctor is
  doing for their pregnancy after stillbirth and start to
  panic that we aren't doing enough, and he reminds me
  that it is just *different* and that we can always ask Dr. B.
- Tells me, often: "We can do this."

● ☾ ●

AS MY BELLY grows, so does the number of questions I
receive. Namely:

Is this your first baby?

How many children do you have?

These seem like such natural questions. Innocent. Safe.
I can't fault the people who ask them, but I always try to
answer honestly no matter how I am feeling or how I imagine they will take the news. When I say that this is my second,
some people just follow up with congratulations, some ask if
I know the sex and if our first is a boy or girl, or how far apart

in age they will be. The phrasing of these questions lets me talk about Reid without talking about his death, and I welcome the opportunity to have a simple conversation about him. Then there are the people who ask how old my first is or where he is at that particular moment. When I share the full truth, I get many different reactions. Some say they are so sorry, and leave it at that. Some look completely gutted and can only turn in the other direction; some look relieved when they think to say, "At least you have this baby now."

To be pregnant again, it feels as if I am being forced to return to *normal*, where all is right in the world and I am happy and grateful and over my loss. I want something to recognize that stillbirth doesn't end after the baby is gone from a family's care, something that acknowledges that it continues and the grief of it infiltrates every aspect of life after that death.

Within my North American, largely nonreligious culture, there's so much discomfort around dealing with grief, and the death that brought it. I don't understand why there is so little to assist us to feel it, carry it, and heal through it, and so much to help us ignore it. Movies that glamorize pain and substances to help numb it, rules put in place to eradicate the possibility of grief talk from our communities, no mention of death or loss or mourning in school systems. I don't know why there is a lack of education about how to have a comforting conversation or give physical and emotional support when someone has suffered a loss. And I don't assume this applies to everyone everywhere, but it seems the real problem is that we don't have a space for authentic grieving at all.

Can we learn from other cultures or religions? How do they grieve? How do they navigate stillbirths, and pregnancy afterward? I do some research and discover that grief varies drastically across cultures—stillbirth-related grief even more so.

Following a stillbirth in Taiwan,[20] families will pray to the gods, pray to their child, burn offerings for them, chant and write scriptures, consult fortune tellers or spiritual mediums, participate in salvation ceremonies for their spirits. Some ceremonies are performed so that a child's spirit might successfully reincarnate. The rituals are done to benefit the deceased child, and to help their immediate family.

In Ethiopia, where infant death rates are some of the highest, babies who are stillborn or die shortly after death are not considered human.[21] They are called "missed babies," thought of as "strangers to families and neighbors." In fact, it is believed that if the stillborn child is mourned, God will bring more misfortune to the family. In one study, an Amharian woman explains that if a woman loses her babies repeatedly, she is called *woldo-bela* (child-killer); it is thought that the deaths were caused by the woman's "evil eye." Sometimes in subsequent pregnancies, parchments with written prayers are fashioned into a necklace to be worn to keep the baby safe until birth. Once the baby is born, before the mother and baby look into each other's eyes, the necklace is placed around the baby's neck.

In Jewish ultra-Orthodox culture, community involvement in death is determined by how many people knew the individual.[22] If a baby dies before birth, very few people participate in the refined mourning rituals. In Judaism, it is common for families to view death as a test of faith from God. This helps them find something positive in their situation. And for some families, even though they know it is a test, they don't understand why the God they know would do this to them.

An American Catholic priest, Thomas Turner, created a ritual to honor babies lost during pregnancy after a woman contacted him to ask if the Catholic Church had any liturgy to honor miscarriage.[23] Caught off guard, he said that he didn't know of any, and the conversation ended. When he recounted this to a religious sister at his parish, she said, "Next time you get a call like that, you make one [a liturgy] up." So he created a mass dedicated to babies who have died, and during it, he asks families to come to the front and light a candle for each baby they have lost in pregnancy. When these masses are held, the whole church is lit up at the front, with families often grabbing more than one candle. It is a way for their seemingly invisible losses to become public ones, and for them to be shared ones, too.

I think of the necklace the Amharian woman was given, the parchment infused with magic meant to keep babies safe. I think of finding a psychic, one who can tell me if I am able to birth boys, tell me if I need to burn ghost money to do so safely. I think of rituals and masses and community-based practices that validate the past in order to support the present.

After the loss of a baby, families turn to intuition, cultural practices, or religious beliefs to help guide them in how they should feel, what they should do. Sometimes, though I think it's rare, these three things align; other times, only two; and then sometimes none of them agree.

If only there were a mediator to help resolve such conflicts, someone who could say, "I see where everyone is coming from. So how about a little bit of intuition for the memory making? A look at what your culture does for the postmortem arrangements? Some religious advice for the mourning?"

"No," I imagine Intuition would respond. "We want the mourning rituals."

"Well, we'd prefer the mourning rituals *and* the memory making," Religion would interject.

"This isn't going to work," Culture would say. "We maintain that babies don't die."

And I think that they might all nod then, finally agreeing. Because this wasn't how it was supposed to go. Babies shouldn't die. But they do, and nothing really makes sense again after that.

● ☾ ●

WHEN I WAS pregnant with Reid, I prepared and researched obsessively. I investigated strollers and car seats and cribs until the space between my eyes throbbed and the screen started to blur. Brittany and I made dates at baby-goods stores and tested out all the available models. We scoured the sale sections of maternity stores. We are planners, so everything was ready long before it needed to be.

With this baby, I already have it all. We have a perfect setup for a little boy. But I can't use any of it. It's Reid's. These things would have been used by Reid's siblings if he hadn't died, but that doesn't help. If he hadn't died, he might not have had siblings. And he *had* died, so I can't insert one baby where I'd spent so much time envisioning another. The nursery isn't just a nursery; it's Reid's room.

We decide to switch rooms. We do this slowly, allowing both the mourning and the enjoyment to come as they please. The moon-and-stars wall decal that Aaron put up last year, the stuffed elephants, the mobile all come down. To go through these things in reverse is more painful than I anticipated. But we have to make room for this second child, and that is a beautiful thing.

It's a comfort to sleep in Reid's room after the switch. His rug and some of his wall hangings remain, so every time my feet touch the floor and my eyes fall upon the walls is a reminder of our time with him.

Now the space that we've created for this new life, this little brother, is uniquely his own. Of course, there are hand-me-downs, carefully selected, separated from the things that will forever remain Reid's. But the beloved child of ours that came before will not overshadow the one that comes after. He will be honored, as we believe he should.

16

"CAN YOU TELL you're having frequent Braxton Hicks?" the nurse asks, studying the strip printing from the monitor.

"Yes." I can feel my stomach tightening. "But they're not painful."

Suddenly, the steady whooshing of the heartbeat slows. I remind myself that monitors slip, babies move, things change. I try to remain calm; I am only thirty-three weeks, at the start of my regular nonstress testing (NST). I am told that when tests begin this early, babies can sometimes misbehave. But when I look to the nurse and notice her brows knit together slightly, I register a hint of concern. "Okay, there was a significant deceleration during one of those last contractions," she says, noting something down on the paper. "This can be normal, but I want to keep you longer just to be sure."

I ask for more ice water and clutch the plastic cup in my hand, sipping nervously. I remembered how my mother told me that all I did was ask for more ice water after Reid was born. I had a vague sense of wanting to give people something to do to help. I also recall being incredibly thirsty.

As part of my care plan for high-risk pregnancies, I'm required to do an NST twice a week from this point onward precisely to pick up abnormalities like this. They involve being hooked up to a contraction and heart-rate monitor and pushing a button whenever you feel the baby move. You're supposed to see a certain number of heart-rate accelerations and a certain number of kicks within twenty minutes. Upon discharge, you're reminded to pay attention to the baby's movements and count their kicks. If you detect reduced movement, it might indicate a problem and give everyone enough time for potentially life-saving interventions.

We monitor the baby for another thirty minutes, through a few more Braxton Hicks, and everything looks normal. An attending doctor concludes the deceleration was likely due to a brief compression of the cord caused by its position and signs off on my test strip. Then I'm discharged and booked for my following NST, a little earlier than originally scheduled. I feel relieved—grateful for the fact that I was in the hospital when it happened.

I start the drive home. Then, just as I leave the hospital, I have another Braxton Hicks. A wave of anxiety comes with it and I pull the car over to the side of the road. I place my hands on my stomach and breathe through it. With no monitors, how can I know the cord isn't compromised again? I wait for another kick. Breathing, rubbing, waiting. Finally, after a few achingly slow minutes, he starts to roll about happily beneath my touch. I feel calm. Peace returns. Then I pull back onto the road and drive home.

● ☾ ●

I'M AT MY parents' house, sitting at their dining-room table with a gestational-diabetes-approved snack of apple slices and almonds in front of me. We are talking about the fact that, for all the significant signs and dreams I've experienced since Reid's death, I never had any premonitions that it was impending. Aloud, I wonder why. My father looks to my mother and she gives him a gentle shrug. He clears his throat to share what he now believes was his.

When I was seven months pregnant with Reid, my father was on a business trip in Toronto. One night, he had what he explains was the most vivid dream he's ever remembered. In the dream, he was holding a baby—our baby. He wheeled him through a forest, headed toward a body of water. As he got closer, he saw that it was a deep blue pool. They sat by the pool, and my father rocked our baby softly in his arms.

Then, the baby transformed into what he could only describe as a being. A beautiful being. And the being leapt off his lap and dove into the pool. My father tried to get out of his chair and dive into the pool after him, but he couldn't move. He cried out to him, frantically wailing for him to come back, reaching toward the water. Then he was startled awake, sweating and weeping in the middle of the night.

He called my mother the next morning to tell her, in a state of complete despair over the fact that in his dream he hadn't been able to save our baby. "It's just a dream," she assured him. "And don't you dare tell Emma." She didn't want to frighten me.

Later that day, my mother received a call from the nanny who had helped raise me and my sisters. She still worked for my parents, helping to manage their household, and I'd asked her to come to our apartment a few times near the end of my pregnancy to help me with a deep clean.

She said she'd had a terrible dream. In it, she saw me clutching my belly, curled up in the corner of a room. I was howling, crying out, "My baby, my baby, my baby." She told my mom the dream seemed so real she needed to call to check that I hadn't given birth, to make sure that everything was okay.

As I hear these stories, I'm left wondering how it works. When these accounts start to accumulate, can they be more than coincidence? Is it even possible to communicate between worlds? And selfishly, I want to know: Why them and not me?

Then I remember my first dream of Reid, the one that was set by the pool of my childhood home. I realize that it was seven months after his birth.

As our due date gets closer, I look for signs that everything will be alright. My monitoring increases: blood tests for my postpartum thyroiditis, specialist clinic appointments for my gestational diabetes, ultrasounds with Dr. B. to check the position of the baby and his cord.

At thirty-seven weeks, at a routine ultrasound with Dr. B., we discover that he has flipped breech. This is not the sign

I was hoping for, and the news shakes me. It means that I can't be induced early, because doctors won't induce breech babies. So that leaves us with a planned cesarean, and since it is already so close to our induction date it will have to be scheduled later. At first, I want to do anything I can to try to flip him. I am ready to buy an ironing board to prop up on the couch and invert myself on, spend my days on my hands and knees, burn pieces of mugwort near my pinky toes in something my acupuncturist calls moxibustion. That evening, a friend messages me to say that she believes that our baby has flipped for a reason. That I should let him have the birth he wants and trust that he knows how to get it. The thought hadn't crossed my mind. Who am I to say what is safest for him?

And then I remember something from a few months ago, in September, when Aaron and I traveled to Galiano Island for our babymoon. We ventured into town and browsed some shops, looking for a few baby things and enjoying the warmth from the softly shining sun. As we were leaving a hardware store a woman stopped us. She looked from my belly to Aaron and then back to me and said, "December 22."

It took me a minute to realize that she was guessing the day our baby would be born. I smiled warmly, knowing my induction was scheduled for three days earlier. "Oh actually, he'll be born on December 19, we know the date."

But she gave me this look—a mixture of mischief and complete seriousness—and firmly said, "No, baby will come on the twenty-second." She made me feel like she was letting me in on a secret, but also poking fun at my certainty. It was such a bizarre encounter with a stranger. But I made a little mental note in case, for some unanticipated reason, our baby had his own plans.

As we wait for a cesarean date, I wonder if it will be scheduled for December 22. And as we try our best to be patient, I let him be. He will flip, or he won't. We will experience labor and a vaginal delivery, or a cesarean. All that matters is that he is safe.

● ☾ ●

IT'S THE MIDDLE of December, a Friday. Aaron and I stand at the street corner and rub our hands together quickly, trying to stay warm as we wait for the light to change. We are expecting the first big snowstorm of the winter on the weekend and we can feel it riding in on the breeze. My Braxton Hicks started to come in stronger and more regular last night, but they disappeared shortly before I went to bed and haven't yet returned. The light has just changed when I feel the slow and steady build of another contraction, but instead of tapering off it sends an ache through my entire body. I reach one hand up to Aaron's shoulder and the other to my belly and shift from one foot to the other as I take a few deep breaths. By the time the lights change again it is over, and I look up to Aaron with a wide grin on my face. *Could this really be happening?*

I try not to get my hopes up. Throughout the pregnancy I've had a recurring dream in which this baby decides to come on his own. I never paid much attention to it, though we have been joking that this baby will probably share a birthday with Derek or Levi, both born in mid-December.

"That'd be cool," Levi would always say whenever we brought it up. Which is fortunate, because today is his birthday.

We get back to our apartment and I've just settled down on the couch for a nap when I notice that the baby's movements are different. Not even twenty-four hours earlier we learned that he had flipped head-down again; our scheduled cesarean was cancelled and induction for labor was rebooked for this Monday. Unable to find the familiar round of his heels now, I think he might have flipped again. My mom is at our place helping with last-minute preparations and when I casually mention this to her, trying (unsuccessfully) to mask my concern, she tells me that I should listen to my instincts and go get checked. I contact Dr. B. and she agrees: we should go to the hospital.

On our way over, at 4:20 PM, I have my first strong contraction. When we get to the hospital parking lot, five minutes later, I have another. Three minutes later, between the car and Admitting, I have a third. They are starting to intensify and by the time we are outside Admitting, I have to stop, double over, and breathe through the contraction.

Just before we walk through the entrance to Labor and Delivery I pause and look up at the wall of tiles with the names of babies who were born in that hospital, and of those who died there too. I find Reid's tile, study his name, and allow the tears to flow before blinking them away.

We are quickly admitted. The nurse who greets us says that she knows our story; she takes us to a curtained-off corner and straps the monitors around my belly right away. *Whoosh. Whoosh. Whoosh.* The sound of his beating heart brings more relief than I expected—I hadn't realized just how nervous I really was. The baby looks great. It turns out he has moved so his back is on the right side of my belly—a position I didn't recognize—and that's why his movements felt different to me. Another thirty minutes of monitoring and we will be clear to go home. But the strip of paper coming out of the monitor confirms that I am definitely having contractions. It's as if my body waited for the trip to the hospital before it felt like it could safely begin the process of bringing this child earth-side.

As I lie on the bed waiting for the OB on call, the waves of tightening start to roll in more frequently and with more intensity. By five o'clock they are two minutes apart and strong. I tell Aaron to let our families know that things might be starting to happen, but because I'm still able to talk and laugh and relax in between contractions, the nurses aren't convinced. Then I get up to use the bathroom and feel a sudden wave of intense pain ripple through me.

I hurry back to bed with Aaron's help, but not before another contraction brings out the first groan. The ones that follow have me breathing so heavily that the nurse comes back in and asks if I want to try the laughing gas. I sense that things are happening quickly, that I could use the help, and I also recognize that accepting this offer will invite the past back in. The memories of using the gas during Reid's birth will attach themselves to the pain I'm experiencing now, but on some level, I need them to.

The nurse wheels in the canister and hands me the mouthpiece. After a quick tutorial, I grip the ribbed hose, place my lips around the tube, and take a long inhale. I'm surprised when I become dizzy, something that hadn't happened before.

As the contraction builds in strength I breathe through the mouthpiece and feel the effects of the gas growing; then when I get to the peak I take the tube out and ride out the rest with controlled breathing. Everything starts to soften. All the while I push as hard as I can against Aaron's hand. The pain is still very much there; I just feel removed from it. And if I close my eyes, take a deep, slow inhale, and surrender to the feeling, I'm able to manage the pain. Later, when I look through our birth photos, I will realize that when I rode the wave of a contraction down from the peak, I was actually smiling.

At 5:20 my dad makes it to the hospital, the first of our family to arrive, though I am too focused on the contractions to have any idea what he says to me. Aaron decides it's time to text our friend and birth photographer, Julie Christine, who is an hour's drive away—he thinks she should probably start the trip, just to be safe. The OB comes in to assess me, asking questions that take forever to get through because I have to stop talking when a new contraction comes. She then checks my dilation. I don't have time to dwell on the discomfort because she laughs and says, "No wonder you're needing the gas. Would you believe me if I told you that you're nine centimeters?"

I laugh out loud too, shocked. Just minutes ago Aaron and I were debating how much more time we should buy for our parking, wondering if an hour would be too long. We definitely aren't going anywhere anytime soon. The OB says my waters are bulging and that we need to get me to a delivery suite as soon as possible.

This is it. I force myself to really absorb what I am feeling, knowing that I'll see this child's face for the first time so soon. I notice exhilaration, terror, peace, and a bit of mourning too. I've spent the better part of the past two and a half years either pregnant or trying to get pregnant. I will miss this season of life, no matter how badly I want the one to come.

As the OB leaves the room and another contraction hits, the monitor shows that the baby's heart rate is decelerating. In the next contraction it gets slower, then slower. And then we lose it completely. A new nurse comes in and moves the monitors around to try to find it again. For the first time since we arrived, I start to cry. I'm brought right back to those minutes before they rolled in the ultrasound machine that pronounced Reid dead, when they were searching for his heartbeat with the very same monitors strapped to my round belly. It has been so long since I've felt this connected to our firstborn son and the pain of losing him. Even through my gratitude for that closeness, grief resurfaces. We soon find the baby's heartbeat and I pull myself together again to prepare for our move upstairs.

"How would you like to manage your pain?" a nurse comes in to ask.

"Well," I start before another contraction hits. It passes; I continue quickly: "I'm assuming there's not time for an epidural?"

"That's right," the nurse says. "Would you like to continue with the gas? Hop in the shower?"

"I'll keep the gas," I say. It's helping; I've found a rhythm with it. Because an epidural was exactly what I needed with Reid's birth, I assumed it would be the same now. But it isn't about me this time—this time there is a living baby to worry about, and he's in a hurry. When I realize this, something changes. The fierceness I can feel rising astounds me. The pain is no longer my enemy but my ally, and it is preparing both my body and my mind to bring new life into this world. I don't think I've ever felt more sure of myself or so capable of anything.

At six o'clock I am guided into a wheelchair to make our trip to the birthing suites upstairs. Off we go, flying through the same halls and over the same bumps I went with Reid, with a nurse pushing my chair and Aaron running close behind, pulling my gas canister with one hand and balancing all of my things in the other—my purse, clothes, water bottle, phone. As we reach the elevator we run into my mom and dad, who tell us my sisters are on the way. I feel like we are living out a scene in a movie, rushing through the halls with more and more people joining in our parade as we go along.

When we finally get to the birthing suite I am hooked up to the monitors again, and we see that the baby is having more significant decelerations. The OB is paged right away, and I know things will move fast now. As we wait, I'm starting to feel numb. My fingers are tingling so intensely that they are completely useless, and my legs are riddled with pins and needles. The nurse assures me that it's just because of my breathing, but I can't believe how severe it is. I'm shaking my hands, trying to get them to feel normal again, when the OB enters the room. After she talks with the nurse and takes a look at the monitor strip she performs a quick exam.

"Alright, Emma. You're fully dilated," she says cheerfully as she pulls off her glove. "It's time to push."

Only I don't feel the urge to push yet. Apparently my waters are preventing the baby from moving down low enough, so it is then suggested that we break them. Seconds before the OB performs the procedure, Julie arrives with her camera already in hand and immediately starts to capture our birth.

I open my eyes and look around the room. There must be ten or fifteen people in here, between the nurses, OBs, pediatrician, Julie, my mom and dad, and Alana and Rebecca, with their partners, Jeremy and Trenton, just on the other side of the door. It definitely wasn't my plan to have my whole family here. Nor did I think I'd be comfortable with so many strangers seeing me at my most exposed—but right now it feels necessary. Since we arrived, I've felt an incredible sense of connectedness to the medical staff. At every turn someone will come up saying that they know our story, read my blog, were there for Reid's birth, or were even working in this hospital the day I was born twenty-six years earlier. We are all on the edge of a precipice together, waiting to witness the birth of this child that means so much to each and every one of us. I sense that they all need to be present for this.

They break my waters with one swift tug and I feel the rush of warm liquid pool beneath me. Immediately—and finally—I feel the urge to bear down, something intense and new to me this time around, with no epidural. The baby's heart rate is still dropping with each contraction, and we are losing it more frequently too. I'm distracted, trying to follow the steady beats, but my ears are ringing loudly from the pain.

Aaron starts talking. "His heart rate is okay," he whispers into my ear. "It's back up now, don't worry. He's doing great. You've got this."

I squeeze my eyes shut and send every ounce of strength I have to my baby. *You're so strong. You can do this*, I say to him over and over in my mind, the power I feel coursing through my body and into our son an extension of what Aaron is sending into me.

The moment I start to push is the moment I wake up. The grief, the numbness, the trauma that I met with Reid—I feel them burn with the fire that grows within me. Feeling everything allows me to *feel everything*. Maybe this physical pain, which I had escaped during Reid's birth, is allowing me to embrace the emotional pain, too.

"We can see his head now," the OB says calmly. "You're almost there." All I can do is ask what color his hair is. Later, it will seem an odd thing to have been preoccupied with. I hear chuckles throughout the room. "It's dark. Very dark." The nurse asks if I want to feel. I nod as I move a trembling hand downward, feeling a soft skull and hair made slippery by the fluids of his home. I am acutely aware that I am touching this precious life for the very first time. I feel the next rush building, the strongest yet.

At 6:44 PM on December 16, 2016, our beautiful son Everett is born screaming.

After exactly twenty-four minutes of pushing—the same amount of time it took to bring his big brother into the world—he is out, sunny-side up, with the cord wrapped around his neck, which the OB quickly clears. As his shoulders emerge the nurse tells me to reach down and grab my baby. Hearing her say those words, looking down to see my son, and placing my fingers around his body brings me right back to those same moments with Reid. I've been here before.

Last time, only one beating heart. This time, two. Last time, I birthed my way into a new world of motherhood in

the silence of my first child. This time, I become a new kind
of mother in the roar of my second. When I pull him up on
my chest and feel his cries ripple through my body the emotions pour into me, and I am transformed, again.

His ribs expand against mine; his fingers stretch and reach
up to grab his ears as they often did during ultrasounds. This
is all new, this heavenly love. It is different from the love I felt
looking at Reid, but both are powerful.

It feels profound to hold Everett just a couple of rooms
down from where we held his older brother. To have met
both of our sons in the same place—a place where we felt
the weight of both life and death so intimately—feels like a
blessing.

Everything that follows Everett's birth is a beautiful dream.
He is measured and weighed—twenty-one inches, six pounds,
twelve ounces—and checked over by the pediatrician. "He's
perfect!" he proclaims. We look down at him, see that he is
the spitting image of his big brother from straight on, and
entirely his own person in profile. Aaron's nose and full lips,
and my dimpled chin and almond-shaped eyes. Then, as I tuck
my finger under his chin to feel how soft his skin is there, he
smiles, revealing a dimple on each cheek.

I've read that when newborns smile, angels are visiting
them. I think about the cord being wrapped around his neck,
reflect back to the ultrasound we had with Dr. B. yesterday,
where it looked like it might have been. As my mind wanders
to these places in these early hours with Everett on my chest,
I feel that Reid played a role in his safe arrival, even if I can't
imagine exactly how.

Aaron's side of our family all arrive within the first hour, entering a room buzzing with the energy of fresh life. They all squeal and hug and wrap me and Aaron in big bear hugs. For a brief moment it is quiet, everyone staring at Everett asleep in my arms. I look from the window, where the snow of the anticipated storm has finally arrived, coming down hard outside, to the scene of warmth at the foot of my bed. It is dreamlike. Then I look to Levi, raise my eyebrows, and say, "Oh, and happy birthday to you too, Levi." We all laugh.

"This is the best gift," he says.

We agree; this day feels like a gift. It feels like the perfect happy ending to our story: the death of a son, followed by the healthy birth of another. A neat and tidy bow I haven't had to fight to tie.

But I should know better, because often the times that feel like endings are really just the latest of beginnings. And what are endings anyway?

17

STAND IN THE elevator, biting my tongue to keep from crying. Fear is penetrating my every thought and action, unlike anything I've ever felt before. I shove it away and try to savor the moment. We are bringing a child home for the very first time. It's a dream we've had for two and a half years—I have to be present. The elevator opens to the eleventh floor and we are suddenly outside our door. The neon-red exit sign above the entrance to the stairs, the fire alarm to the left of us, our apartment to the right. Everything is the same, but it all looks different.

Aaron lets us in, drops the bags at the entrance, then turns around and brings Everett over the threshold. The lights on our Christmas tree are shining and the halls smell of cinnamon and cloves. I can see someone has turned on the little lamp on the side table in the nursery, and it is glowing in anticipation.

Aaron unbuckles Everett's tiny body from the car seat and hands him to me. I bounce and sway and take him through each room, introducing him to his home. *This is the front hall, here to the left is the bathroom, straight ahead there is where your nursery is.* I coo and bounce and sway, coo and bounce and sway. *This is your parents' room, the living room, the dining area.* His eyes go wide, seemingly in awe. When the tour is over I suggest to Aaron that we attempt a diaper change.

In the nursery, we sift through our stash of diapers only to find that we don't have the right size. We have ones and twos but no Ns, for newborns. I hadn't anticipated he'd be so small.

"We could call my mom?" I offer. But then thinking aloud, "Though it'll be a while by the time she gets here with them."

"Would you be okay with me heading down to the drugstore real quick?" Aaron asks.

Either we all go to the store—with a two-day-old baby and a very unsteady mother—or he goes by himself, leaving the two-day-old baby and unsteady mother on their own. Aaron is probably thinking much more clearly than I am, so I agree.

The minute Aaron leaves I have to pee. But when I stand up, Everett still in my arms, I feel a gush between my legs. A clot has passed, and I cringe feeling the blood soak through my adult diaper. I grab the cushioned change pad from the dresser with one hand, balance Everett in the crook of my left arm, and waddle to the bathroom. I place the change pad on the counter and slowly lower Everett to it, then strip down. I'm wearing a onesie, so it all has to come off. There is blood everywhere. I laugh. Then, having been startled awake, Everett starts to scream. I put one hand on him to soothe him and reach under the cupboard to grab a pad and a new diaper, only to realize that all of my postpartum care is in our hospital bags down the hall. Everett is completely distraught and I'm trying to recall what I've read about leaving newborns briefly unattended on change pads as I bleed into the toilet. Unable to think, I scoop him into my arms and sing the one lullaby I know, "Hush Little Baby," as I hold him to my chest. He stops crying and the bleeding tapers. I lean back against the lid of the toilet.

Aaron comes through the door shortly after with a smile plastered on his face, holding up a frozen pizza, chocolate milk, and Cinnamon Toast Crunch. I hadn't asked for any of those things, but somehow he knew they were exactly what I was craving. But then he sees the blood on the floor, and me naked, and the two of us on the toilet in the bathroom. Struck with panic, he drops the smile. I laugh so hard the tears I'd fought to keep back come anyway. What a vision we must be.

"Never leave us again!" I shout.

We've made it through our first parenting hurdle, and after Everett is put in a clean diaper and a freezer meal is defrosted and laid out on our coffee table, we make our way over to the couch.

Then the anxiety returns. I thought I'd felt anxiety during pregnancy, but it was nothing compared to what I'm experiencing now. I watch Everett's chest moving up and down, notice his fragile body shake with the effort, and wonder how it is possible that we are solely responsible for his life now. There will be no more weekly ultrasounds, no more NSTs. This is it. And it feels so terribly wrong. All of it. Where is the happy, sleepy ease I've read about?

I become obsessed with watching his breathing. From the CPR course we took as a family a couple of weeks earlier, I know all it takes is thirty seconds or less for a child to go blue in the face when their oxygen supply is cut off. Any longer than that and they could lose consciousness. Then they'd very quickly go pale. Then brain damage. Death wouldn't be far behind. So every thirty seconds I look in his direction. If Aaron sleeps, I'm awake watching him. If Aaron is watching him, I am still awake too, because I can't trust anyone else to watch him as closely as is necessary. I know about postpartum anxiety and I wonder if that is what I'm experiencing. I make a mental note to mention it during the public health nurse's visit the next day.

We so badly want to handle the first few days at home on our own, but by the second day I have to call my mom. She is over in thirty minutes. She brings food, helps us tidy the apartment, and finally convinces us she'll watch Everett sleep while we take a nap. She knows me; she'll watch him like I need her to. Besides, she keeps babies alive.

I wake up after two hours and feel like a new person. It's the first time I've slept in three days. But I still feel anxious. My mom leaves us to have dinner with a promise to return tomorrow to help out again. We're slicing rosemary and olive oil bread as we wait for our tomato soup to cool. It is the same meal we had as we waited for labor to begin with Reid. Aaron is browsing Netflix, asking how long I think it might be before I feel comfortable enough that we can all sleep at the same time, and Everett is sleeping to our right. Thirty seconds. I look over to him. My spoon hits the floor. I lunge toward his body.

"Aaron. He's blue." I speak calmly at first, picking him up and trying to rouse him. When he doesn't move I start to scream. "He's blue!" I howl. "Oh god, Aaron, he's blue!"

I repeat it over in my mind as I run with him into the nursery, where the lighting is the best. *He's blue, he's blue, he's blue.* I shout at Aaron to follow me. In the light I can see something is horribly wrong. His forehead is streaked through with blue veins and his lips are dark. I rip the loose swaddle off him, tear my own shirt off, and place him on my chest, rubbing his back with a panicked strength.

My heart beats through my chest. I remember that bunnies sometimes get so scared, their hearts beat so fast that they just drop and die. I wonder, momentarily, if there is any real possibility of that happening to me. Then I think it is such a peculiar thing to be thinking in this moment. But I keep rubbing, all the while staring at Aaron's face, which is frozen with shock. Suddenly, a cry. My whole body surrenders to a tremble as I watch his color return.

I feel crazy. Aaron didn't see any of it, it happened so quickly. What seemed like ages was only a few seconds, he says. And as I start to recount what I saw, I become less and less sure. It can't be true. My mind must've made it all up. There is a pink, screaming, wiggling baby on my chest, probably very mad at the fact that he is being struck on his back.

Should we call the nurse hotline? Should we take him to the hospital? Should we feed him? My body won't stop shaking. The familiar panic rises, a panic I haven't felt in twenty months. Aaron feels the crisis is averted.

"Look, he seems completely fine. Let's finish dinner," he suggests. "We'll feel better after we eat."

But I can't let it go. "Let's call Micaela?" I ask.

Aaron agrees. I pull out my phone and hand it to him, unable to talk myself. There is no answer, so we try again.

Then twice more, and there is still no answer. I tell him to call the next nurse I know, Brittany. As the phone rings I try to push aside the fact that she is the last person I talked to before we found out Reid died.

I hear her voice on the other end. "Hello?"

"Hi Brittany, it's Aaron."

"Aaron?" she asks, clearly confused that he is speaking from my number. "Is everything okay?"

"Well, no. We're home—" He pauses to put the phone on speaker. "Emma thinks Everett went blue. We are wondering what we should do."

She has Aaron recount everything I told him very carefully. As it so happens, she is at work right now, so she excuses herself to go consult with the attending pediatrician.

"Okay. I know this isn't what you want to hear. If it truly was a blue spell then you should take him in," she explains tenderly. "It was likely just that he got himself in a funny position that cut off his airway, but they'll want to monitor him for a few hours anyway. You'll go to Emergency at the children's hospital."

Aaron nods, says thank you. I start to make a mental list of what we need to leave the house. Diapers, a change of clothes, pants for me.

"And Aaron?"

"Yeah?"

"I'm so sorry. Emma will never sleep again, will she?" She pauses. "Please keep me posted."

Aaron asks again if I'm sure we should go in. "Is it the right call? He'll be exposed to so much there."

He is worried, and so am I, but it isn't a question anymore. We will call my mom; we will all go to the ER. Everything moves slowly and methodically from this point. I hand Everett to Aaron and go into the bathroom to brush my teeth. I think about putting dry shampoo in my hair but instead decide to braid it quickly down my back. I put on clothes, taking care to remember the pants. Aaron calls my mom and asks her to meet us at the hospital. I grab medical documents and pack a bag for Everett.

In the car, I sit in the back beside him with my fingers pressed against his chest as we drive back to the hospital we left just two days ago. My thoughts focus in on his breathing, which sounds labored, small, and raspy. But what does normal infant breathing sound like?

As we pull up to the Emergency parking lot my mom is waiting for us, lit in silhouette by the bright hospital signs behind her.

"Be careful," she says, "there's black ice everywhere."

Later, we learn that the hospital had run out of salt that evening. People had been fighting over it for days, in the midst of the snowstorm, and they had finally used up the last of their reserves. So we skate across the parking lot, and with each step I take I slide a little, feeling the pain of each stretch ripple through my tender muscles.

"Don't drop him," I repeat to Aaron, over and over again. I have visions of him flying across the lot, the car seat tumbling from his grasp, Everett's tiny skull hitting the icy pavement.

When we finally make it to the sidewalk we walk toward the entrance. Slowly at first, and then I set the pace at a run. We burst through the sliding glass doors to find a packed waiting room. I pull the medical papers from my bag and run up to Admitting. The nurse is with another patient and I pace. *Why is it taking so long?* I feel like I'm going to be sick.

I'm not sure what comes over me, but I suddenly run back to where my mom and Aaron are sitting waiting with Everett in the car seat, the cover still on.

"Is he okay? Check on him," I bark at Aaron.

Aaron peers into the car seat. "I think—" His face sinks.

I leave my body at this point, like I did in this same hospital twenty months ago, watching everything unfold from above. I watch as Aaron rips the cover off and wrenches on the buckles. I watch myself run toward the nurse, screaming for her to get help. I watch the heads in the waiting room turn in our direction. I watch as our son is pulled from the car seat, pale, lifeless, and cold. I watch Aaron hand him over to the nurse. I watch as we all run down the hall, the nurse shouting orders and calling for doctors. I watch as Everett's limbs dangle below her hands. I notice his head is at an awkward angle and his mouth is slightly ajar, and I think how very similar he looks to Reid. Dead, but mine. But dead.

Everett is thrown onto a table and I lose sight of him in a sea of doctors and nurses working to resuscitate him. Time goes by. Seconds? Minutes? Then, "I have a pulse!" a physician shouts.

They throw phrases back and forth: *Breathing is raspy. Unstable. Need a urine sample. Let's sedate him.*

My mom, Aaron, and I huddle in an embrace at the edge of the room.

I text Micaela:

We're in the ER.

Minutes later, Micaela appears. She is on shift in the PICU upstairs. She runs over to us, the yellow hospital gown flapping out behind her, and sobs into my arms. After giving each of us a hug she goes over to one of the nurses in the crowd by Everett's bed and embraces her too.

My mother and I stand by Everett's side, and I stroke his face as my father did mine when I was small. Down the forehead toward the brows, then along each brow from the center out toward the edges. As I do I repeat the same words he always said to me, "I love you more than the sun and the moon and the stars, more than the whole universe." To my right, at the head of his gurney, is a young man, younger than me. He squeezes the bag pumping air into Everett's lungs.

"Are you good? Do you need a coffee? A chair?" my mom asks him, completely serious.

"No, ma'am," he replies. "I'm fine."

"You're sure?" she presses. "Because you've got my grandson's life in your hands there."

I want to laugh, but I am sure it isn't meant to be funny.

Twenty minutes go by. Someone says that nothing has changed, he isn't breathing steadily without assistance, they need to intubate. We're asked to step back and we watch as the sea of blue scrubs and white coats engulfs him once again.

● ☾ ●

OVER AND OVER again we repeat to the doctors, "Our first son was stillborn." It isn't meant to help them with a diagnosis, but surely it will help them see the mistake here. It is as if to say: *This can't be happening, you see, because lightning doesn't strike twice. We were promised.* And it is true. We have been promised by every doctor. We have been through our life-altering event. So we say it to anyone who asks what happened. "Our first son was stillborn," is how we always begin. We watch their faces light up, in the way that only a medical professional's face can light up at that news. "And did they ever find out—" They don't need to finish their question. "Yes," I say. "A true knot in his umbilical cord." They offer their condolences, and I know their faces only fall because their breadcrumb, their possible clue, has been swept away by my words.

Aaron looks gaunt. His head hangs low and his hair sticks straight up from running his hands through it so much. A NICU doctor commends us, says, "You probably just saved his life by bringing him in as quickly as you did." Aaron just shakes his head and says that it was all me.

I've known Aaron for nearly a decade now, and it's clear to me what he's thinking: that things might have gone differently had we made a different choice, perhaps the one he'd suggested where we waited to go to the hospital, or didn't go at all. He had only done what he does best, which is think through things logically, weigh the supposed risks against any possible benefits.

I know this because I'm thinking the same thing, that I so easily could have failed. What if I had nursed Everett before leaving or spent a little more time on my hair or finished my meal? What if I hadn't been watching him as obsessively as I had? What if Brittany hadn't answered the phone? So many *what ifs*; it is strange to be on the other side of them. Not thinking of the one thing we could have done differently that could have saved a life, but the one thing we could have done differently that could have ended one.

A discussion takes place about where to put us. Technically, given that Everett was discharged from the hospital and went home, he belongs in the pediatric intensive care unit, not the neonatal one. But the PICU is on discharge to Alberta, the next province over, meaning any new patients coming to them have to be sent there. However, given that Everett was only home two days, the rules and regulations could be blurred slightly. NICU might be able to accept him if the department head signs off on it. All I know is, Micaela disappears for a while, and when she comes back we are being transferred to isolation in the NICU.

Because the cause of Everett's "episodes," as they are calling them, are unknown, they have to consider a virus as a possibility. He must be placed in isolation until testing proves otherwise. We are given a private room at the back of the crowded nursery, in one of the procedure rooms. Tents and a gowning station are set up and we are instructed to robe and mask ourselves when coming and going. Medical professionals have to cover up completely: they wear full face masks with plastic visors, yellow gowns that flow down to their ankles, and thick white gloves that go over the sleeves up to their elbows. As these costumed figures float around me, I sit topless by Everett's incubator, trying to figure out how to manage a breast pump. I pump until my nipples crack and bleed, and still, I keep on pumping.

None of it feels real. I think that helps.

I text Dr. B. with the news. When she arrives only a few hours later, she immediately looks through Everett's file and speaks with the doctors. I can tell she is smiling behind her mask as she talks, but her eyes have a less cheerful look, one that I recognize. I wonder if she is looking for someone to blame. She got Everett into our arms and made good on her promise—a promise she worked nine long months to support—and yet here we are, four days after his birth, relying on machines to keep him alive.

I mention the woman who drew Everett's blood for his newborn testing, about how she wore a mask, saying she had a cold.

"I'm an aunt," she'd said. "And I know that's no way for anyone to start life." We laughed, thanked her for being so considerate. She coughed, touched her mask briefly, went back to her work, squeezing blood from his heel.

Dr. B. relays this to Everett's team.

"I should have requested someone else to draw his blood," I confess.

"This isn't your fault," she says. She might believe this, but I'm not sure that everyone does. Last night during rounds, one of the doctors on Everett's case announced, while looking at me, that they should be testing for toxicity, considering parental factors. My greatest fear is that I have done this, so I look the doctor in the eye and tell him to run whatever tests they need. I tell him to save our son. These tests all come back normal, the doctor who ordered them looks slightly disappointed to tell me.

Dr. B. hugs me before she leaves, offers up her couch at her home across the street should I need to sleep, and texts me often. I still rely on her, and she knows it. Though the situation is out of her hands now, I still feel that she can make it all okay. If not her, then who?

Sitting in the NICU, praying for Everett to gain the strength to wake up, I feel betrayed by the God I thought was good. What do I need to do to get my son back? If I'm loud enough for long enough, will He grant me my wish? If I pray with all I have, if I ask my thousands of followers on social media to join me, will He concede? And if Everett's life is saved, what does that mean? I've prayed for the lives of both my sons. I want Everett, but I wanted Reid too.

Right now I don't believe God is good. Honestly, am I sure I even believe in Him at all?

● ☾ ●

AFTER TWO DAYS in intensive care, Everett still hasn't opened his eyes. I keep asking the nurses if they are sure they aren't giving him any sedatives. They keep assuring me they aren't, looking every bit as nervous as I feel.

When we asked his doctor how his spinal tap procedure went, she said, "It went too well, actually," and shook her head as she removed her visor and mask.

"What do you mean?" Aaron asked.

"Most babies cry and protest and have to be held down," she explained. "Your son didn't even flinch."

We still don't know what to make of this news. And now, his heart rate is continuing to drop. From the hundreds to the nineties to the eighties. The alarms sound when the lower threshold is passed; nurses check his vitals, then adjust their parameters another ten below the last. I ask when they will stop adjusting the limits on that machine and instead do something to help him, and they respond that they usually intervene when an infant's heart rate drops into the sixties.

We are in the seventies now. I am staring at the screen, watching it change from seventy-five beats per minute to seventy-eight and then down to seventy-three. Suddenly, sixty-nine. Alarms start sounding. Then his number is back in the mid-seventies again and they stop. This dance continues, and as it does Micaela enters the room. I am panicked. "They said that they'll do something when his heart rate drops into the sixties, and it's doing that now. But no one is doing anything! I don't understand!" I tell her.

"That's strange, it shouldn't be that low," she says. She checks a few of his monitors and leaves the room to speak with his team outside the door. When she comes back, she says, "The NICU operates differently than us, and I don't really understand why they make certain decisions. But Everett isn't fitting into one specific box, so they're just waiting."

I look at the machine that's breathing for him, listen to its steady tones, and try to find assurance in the fact that it is keeping him alive while we wait. What exactly are we waiting for? More test results? His numbers to change? Death, perhaps? I get ready to pump again, and do the one thing I can while I wait.

A few hours later, Everett's heart rate unexpectedly stabilizes. Then, finally, he opens his eyes. I jump to his side, stroke his hair and whisper, "Hush now, everything is okay, Mama's here." Tears stream down my cheeks and I take a video to send to our family.

As I sit in the chair beside his incubator, watching nurses enter and exit the room in their alien suits, listening to the hum and beep of the machine that breathes for him, I try to make sense of it. Then I realize the date: it is December 22. I think back to that woman from our babymoon who said that Everett would come on the twenty-second. She was so sure. Now I wonder if what she sensed, in some impossible way, wasn't that he would come to us on the twenty-second: maybe it was the day he would come back.

● ☾ ●

WE ARE STILL under isolation; more tests need to be run to rule out other possible viruses, but the holidays are making things move slowly. They want us out of the general NICU bay, though, so when a suitable room becomes available in a new wing, called South, we are moved there. The process makes me nervous. A respiratory therapist has to bag Everett, so they can disconnect him from the ventilation machine, and a team of specialists wheel the rest of the equipment down the halls as we walk.

The transfer goes smoothly, and I cry when the charge nurse tells me the room is connected to a bathroom with a shower. She hands me some scratchy, bleached hospital towels and I take my first shower in days, sob under the hot water as steam fills the room. After, we set up a thin foam mattress underneath the sinks in the room; this is where Aaron and I will live.

The NICU is dated, not family-centered, and it's not standard protocol to allow parents or caregivers to stay with their babies. They are building a new NICU as part of the current hospital renovation. But until it's finished, they're not really set up for that situation, and they keep trying to get us to leave.

Later, someone finally asks our nurse, Sam, who is an old high school friend, to convince us to sleep at home. They are concerned that we need a break. I explain that I understand we must be an inconvenience, but the most traumatic thing I can think of, besides having Everett die too, is going home with empty arms again. I'm not sure I'd survive it. And if Everett did die, I'd never forgive myself for spending that time away from him. She must have advocated for us to be allowed to stay, because no one tries to make me leave again after that.

On day three in intensive care, the doctors suggest trying to remove Everett's breathing tube. Though he still uses the machine for breathing support while he is asleep, he is independent while awake, trying to pull the tubes out on his own. They don't want him to start to rely on it, have it become his norm so he gets lazy. I am sleeping as they start to do it, and Aaron shakes me awake mere seconds before they remove the tube. When they do, Everett lets out a hoarse little cry, and I am grateful for the noise. He looks like he has gone to battle; red patches are left from the tape holding the tubes in place, and putty from the brain monitor leaves his hair tacky.

Afterward, his blood oxygen levels continue to drop below the lower threshold and his breathing pauses for significant moments while he sleeps. But no serious interventions are needed. When the alarms go off overnight or when he naps, Aaron or I run over and rouse him, bringing his levels up within range as he wakes in response. What we need is time. Time to run tests, time to see if the CO_2 levels that build up in his blood overnight will return to normal on their own.

He's had a spinal tap, blood tests, biochemistry profiles, chromosomal analysis, ultrasounds, X-rays, EEGs, ECGs, polysomnograms, an MRI. A handful of these things come back with abnormal results, but none can give us any answers for why this happened. No one can even tell us what these abnormal results mean. Eventually, some will improve, though some of them won't.

Aaron's spirits lift considerably after Everett finally regains consciousness. He talks to him. He helps with every single tube feed, and then bottle when he's cleared for them, and changes every single diaper too. He disappears, then returns with a decaf latte for me to consume post-pump. He is there for all of the doctors' morning rounds, asking questions and gathering information while I sleep underneath the sink. What a difference hope makes. With hope, we become a team. We could not endure this alone, but together we support our fragile family through.

On Christmas Day in the NICU, my breasts are so swollen and covered in red welts that when Sam walks in and sees me pumping, she orders me to go down the hall to the women's hospital. I don't want to go.

I leave Everett with Aaron. My mom and I make the same walk I did after our diagnostic ultrasound after Reid passed, but this time in reverse.

We get to Admitting and I stop in my tracks. The nurse behind the desk is Hilary. Hilary, who couldn't find Reid's heartbeat that Good Friday. And here I am seeing her again for the first time since, on Christmas Day.

She doesn't recognize me. I tell her that I hope it isn't busy and that our NICU nurse told us it was a good time to come. I haven't been away from Everett's side for more than fifteen minutes at this point, I say.

She looks at me and snarks in frustration that she doesn't know who told me that but she can't guarantee anything quick and that births get priority. I flush and instead of trying to explain what I meant, I only say, "Of course."

Another nurse, who remembers me from Reid, admits us and says not to worry. She doesn't think Hilary realized who I am, nor how we are connected. I thank her for saying so and wipe away the tears.

In the waiting area, I sit directly below Reid's tile. My mom goes off to get me a sandwich so I can eat while I wait. Then Hilary appears from behind a pillar. She is biting her lip, the same way she had as she'd maneuvered the Doppler, and I notice her hand reach down to rub her swollen belly. I hadn't realized she was pregnant.

"Emma? I'm so sorry," she begins. "I didn't recognize who you were right away. But I have thought of you so much over the years."

We both start to cry. She asks if she can give me a hug and I stand up to meet her embrace.

"And now you're in the NICU with your second son. It's not fair."

I thank her, and I tell her he has taken a positive turn.

Then I am called into the examining room. Apparently it is nothing more than severely clogged ducts; the doctor tells me to massage them in a hot shower and, if possible, to push to begin breastfeeding soon.

As I leave I pause before Hilary and meet her gaze. "Thank you for coming up and saying something to me," I say. She smiles and so do I, and I walk back toward the room where Everett is sleeping.

18

W E HAVE BEEN living in the hospital with Everett for two and a half weeks now. In the procedure room, we took shifts sleeping in the chair next to his incubator. In South, we slept on the thin foam mattress wedged under the sink in his room. When his isolation was finally lifted in the first week of January, we were moved out of the private room and into a general bay. Again, the only place to sleep is in a chair beside him, and now that I'm breastfeeding I'm the one who stays, while Aaron sleeps in the waiting room, though he's not technically allowed.

Eventually, a new doctor comes on the team and is willing to admit that there are likely no answers to be found. Everett's near death, and his current improved health, cannot be explained medically. Now that he is, by all appearances and testable standards, stable, this doctor is convinced that the best thing possible for all of us will be to go home.

We agree with him: we need to go home. We aren't sure we are ready, but we can't stay here either.

● ☾ ●

"WHAT DO YOU need to go home and feel safe?" The social worker is studying my face.

What do I need? "I need someone to tell me that everything will be okay," I say. "But you can't do that, can you?"

She shakes her head no, writes something down, and has just opened her mouth to speak when I cut her off. "The only reason Everett is alive is because I watched him obsessively. How can I ever take my eyes off him when that was what saved his life?"

She is silent.

My mother once told me a story about my Nana, my father's mother—about a moment from my father's own life.

He was a teenager, about to venture out with two friends to go fishing. Before he left she held him close and frantically pleaded with him not to hitchhike. She'd never pleaded with him like that before—it was as if she had become an entirely different mother. My father shrugged and told her that of course they wouldn't, they had their own ride, then skipped out the door with his rod over his shoulder.

He did hitchhike. They got back from their fishing trip and stopped at the ranch of one friend, about halfway between where they were camping and Williams Lake. The other friend and my dad had a scheduled ride home the next day, but because they were early and wanted to see the famous Williams Lake Stampede, they decided to hitchhike the rest of the way. They stuck out their thumbs for five cars, turning down one ride that would have left them with thirty more miles at the end. The sixth car passed them slowly, and they jumped up to flag it down. Abruptly, the driver stopped. When they got a look at his face they realized that it was a man they'd helped with a flat tire at the beginning of the trip; he had stopped because he recognized them and wanted to return the favor.

They got in that pickup truck and filled the back up with their catches from the day. His friend sat on a metal toolbox in the back; my dad sat in the truck bed beside him. At the last minute, the friend asked to switch places. He was feeling unwell, wondering if he might feel better if he could recline. My dad took his place and off they went.

When the driver turned a corner, the pickup truck flipped. Thrown from the back, my dad landed on the hard edge of the toolbox he'd been sitting on, corner to spine, shattering the bones and then the cord beneath them. That was the accident that paralyzed him from the waist down. A string of precisely timed events and split decisions altered everything for him. And they are the only reason I exist at all.

There have been other moments when my Nana did or said things that could not be explained. Like the day our family cat, Clancy—a beautiful orange tabby—had to be suddenly put down. That afternoon, after he was gone, we received a notepad from her in the mail that she'd sent weeks earlier. The pages were shaped like a cat, with an orange tabby printed on each one, fifty of them piled high.

Then there were times when her intuition was off. She'd call our home in the middle of the night in a panic, shouting into my mom's ear, "Where's Ricky? Is he okay?"

I used to think she was crazy. Sometimes when she'd call the house I would ignore it, not wanting to bear the brunt of her frightened tales. But a mother's intuition is strong. She isn't crazy; what happened to her was crazy.

Will I be the same, years down the road? Will I think that a nightmare is intuition and ring up Everett's home to yell in his spouse's ear too?

I know now that what I experienced leading up to Everett's episodes was intuition, and what I felt in the room with that social worker was fear. The two feel so similar. But that sense that Everett would not be okay was different. That I had taken a CPR course, that I needed to monitor his sleep, that I brought him to the hospital so quickly were all things I did because of Reid, because he died. Not because of anxiety, or at least not entirely, but because of a change in the way I viewed what was important and what was not—because of the lessons his brief life taught me, the instincts that all the experiences that ensued have allowed me to refine. In the way that I no longer lean solely on the false comforts of what statistics and science and majorities say are most likely, but also look to what I innately feel to be true.

Reid likely had a far greater role in everything than I'll ever know in this life. I don't believe he was actually in the room with me—though, gosh, I did feel him there. But this feeling, this intuition, felt God-given. This presence that was so beyond my own took over, leading the way. That's the only way I can describe it—so similar to that prophetic light I felt during and shortly after Reid's birth. People put their babies down to rest in separate rooms all the time, but I knew that I couldn't. Ultimately, I cannot pretend to know the whys. All I can do is tell the truth and lean into my faith where there are unknowns. And what is true is this: Everett is not here *instead* of Reid, but he is here *because* of him.

In the end, we receive no official diagnosis. After nearly three weeks in the NICU, the doctor who will ultimately discharge us concedes to call it a BRUE (brief resolved unexplained event). He suspects that Everett's combination of exaggerated periodic breathing (which still persists) and episodes of apnea (which he still has) met with a virus (their best guess), producing a perfect storm that caused him to stop breathing, and then not know how to start again. Maybe the specific positions had contributed to that perfect storm: he had fallen asleep in a rocker at home, was in a car seat in the ER waiting room. Either way, he had been very sick, that had been clear, and he has gotten much better. That may be all we ever know.

● ☾ ●

I WEEP INTO the scratchy brown hospital paper towel.

We were discharged officially this morning, but they aren't rushing us. We put Everett in the car seat and it looks wrong—different from the way it did yesterday during his required car seat test, when he was hooked up to monitors to make sure his tiny body could handle the position—and the nurse doesn't know how to help and none of the staff we have come to know are there. I'm crying, asking for help, anxious. No, it isn't even anxiety. It is debilitating panic badly camouflaged as such. The car seat—the car seat that held him lifeless. We ask if we can carry him to the car and put him in that car seat at the very last minute. They say we can't. An insurance issue if we trip.

So we move hastily and I sob and grab the paper towel from the dispenser, try to pass it off as tissue paper. And then we run into the night custodian I spent these past weeks getting to know. She is thrilled to see us and looks in at the car seat to get a glimpse of Everett. Then, seeing my tears, she says, "Be happy! This is happy!" I cry some more and say that they are happy tears. But no part of me is happy. We fought for this moment, desperately wanted it, and then to *actually* leave the safety and security of the monitors and doctors— well, that changes everything.

I don't remember the car ride home.

Then I'm stripping down to my skin at the door (germs) and yanking him out of the car seat (PTSD) and collapsing on the couch (exhaustion). My mom comes in shortly after with groceries and clean laundry in hand and an overnight bag to spend the night. I'm relieved and shocked to be home with my baby. After it all, here I am. Home. With a baby. Home with Everett. But now what?

For the next two weeks, as we wait for more results of more tests, night nurses watch Everett as he sleeps in his nursery— so that we can sleep too—and keep me company as I nurse him every three hours. For the next two weeks, I also have nightmares. I wake up from the same horrible dream where I see it again: Everett's pale blue face and dark lips. But I see it in a thousand different ways. He is in bed with us and we fall asleep and suffocate him; we drop him as we walk him through the halls; he chokes on milk and never recovers. I wake up in a full sweat, or sometimes I don't wake up at all but instead bolt up in bed, still deep inside my nightmare, and search frantically for the child that isn't there. Aaron has to gently fold me in his arms and calm me back to sleep.

Our world revolves around doctors' appointments and development programs and NICU discharge follow-ups. Then, of course, there are the germs. His doctors' main worry is that because he never received a diagnosis, we can only speculate. This means that we have to cover all of our bases. The biggest fear is that if he gets sick again, the same thing will happen. As long as he appears to have underlying issues of centrally triggered apnea, while he is so young, it is a concern.

Germs are our enemy. Visitors have to wear masks in our home; when we go out I wear Everett close to my body so strangers keep their distance; anyone who has been in contact with anyone (who has been in contact with anyone) who was sick has to stay away for at least a week before we can entertain the idea of them visiting.

This plays right into my neuroses. When I was a child, the need to be clean devoured me. A nurse had come to our class to teach us how to wash. We scrubbed our hands with special foaming soap and then held them under a black light, which showed the germs that remained. Mine lit up like the Milky Way. After, I began washing them obsessively. I'd accidentally touch a table and then have to run to the bathroom to scrub. I'd rub my hands so raw they would bleed.

I feel much the same after leaving the NICU with no diagnosis. We are told to keep Everett safe, to keep him clean.

I am on high alert, always. A woman sneezes in the corner of a shop and I turn abruptly on my heels and walk-run toward the door. An elderly man peers into my babywearing wrap to get a closer look and I lunge back, ready to swat away a hand should it attempt a touch. I look on at the couples in restaurants who hand their infants off to the waitstaff to be cuddled, baffled at how they could be so careless.

Then I realize, with gut-wrenching clarity, that what I am witnessing is normal behavior. We are, in fact, the abnormal ones. Going on living life preparing for the fact that our son *may* have a life-threatening condition that could cause him to stop breathing without warning. Ready to draw our CPR training out from the backs of our brains. We have nothing to go by. No rules, just precautions. I wrestle constantly with myself about the potential risks and benefits of any situation.

Everett's pediatrician warns against intimate social situations. "Best to limit it to the people he's already been exposed to," he says. But friends (who become strangers) don't understand why family can see him but they cannot. Our nonunderstanding of everything doesn't help. We can't give answers. There are none.

Later, upon testing his organic acids levels, we discover that one is extremely high. The organic acids are part of what is called the Krebs cycle, which creates the energy needed to sustain all processes necessary to maintain life. Breathing, for example. When this particular imbalance is present in babies, blue spells have been observed. But these babies are usually not expected to live long and have other symptoms, our doctor explains. They will look different, have physical deformities, serious complications with basic physiological functions. "Your child," he says, "does not present with any of these. If this doesn't resolve, he will be the first baby I've seen with this condition without them." Perhaps instead, he suggests, whatever made him ill affected this level and aggravated his already present symptoms. It is possible—these results are the only medical evidence that indicate a virus.

The levels are all normal now. We may never know why.

Months later, we are still doing studies. Polysomnograms continue, and will repeat once a year until the results either tell us something new or come back normal. We spend the night in the outpatient clinic with the respirology team at the children's hospital. Everett is hooked up to an EEG and an oxygen pulsometer and a strap is fastened around his chest to test his breathing. I sleep on the single mattress beside his crib and crawl in to nurse him back to sleep when he wakes. Aaron sleeps in an empty medical bed in a room next to us.

Each test is better. Apneic episodes dropping from the hundreds to the tens to, now, just above the normal upper limit of a few per night. But the apnea is still always there. His respirologist is surprised but not worried by these results. If he did these studies on one hundred healthy babies, he says, one of them would likely have the same results. But he offers to keep testing until he can one day tell us things are "normal" by the test's standards.

So do we live in a constant state of readiness? Alert and prepared for anything? What is the difference between stifling him and keeping him safe? How far do we go?

● ☾ ●

A MILLION TINY, specific choices had to be made for me to end up with a child attached to my breast, rocking him to sleep. When I transfer Everett to his crib, I watch his chest rise and fall. I place the monitor on his foot and stare at the numbers of his heart rate and oxygen levels; I watch them rise and fall too. I love him, I love him, I love him. I cannot imagine anyone but him. I want to wrap him up and protect his life at all costs. But one day, we will need to stop monitoring him, and this will be a choice. One day, there will be no more tests, though likely no certainties either.

I don't notice until later that the choices required of us don't always look like action. Sometimes, we don't have a choice. Sometimes, choices are made for us. And when they are, the choice we have is in our attitude or outlook or response.

What I want, I finally understand, is for someone to tell me that we have done all we can, and that it will still be enough when we stop searching—waiting—for answers. That our choice to lead with hope is the right one. No one can promise me that, as no one can rightfully promise lightning, or tragedy, wouldn't strike more than once. But when that doctor made that promise after Reid died, it was what I needed to hear. I needed courage to believe in something good, even if he was vowing something he couldn't guarantee. And that is life. Fragile. Unpredictable. Precious. We must hold the things we love dearest with open hands because none of it is permanent. All that we know is that everything we understand and love and embrace changes.

19

KNOCK TWICE ON her door. I hear her run to answer, and when she opens it her long, black hair is still billowing out behind her. She wears it shaved close to her skull in a strip above her right ear, the way she did the last time I saw her.

Teresa welcomes me into her home, and I pause at her window, take in the view of the mountains capped with snow. She looks out at them too, says, "The elders are wearing their ceremonial cloaks this morning." Then she leads me to a clear space on her living-room floor. It's adorned with jewel-toned fabrics, a deck of cards and a line of rocks displayed at one end. Ready for the ceremony she generously offered to gift me a year ago now.

She tells me it's a sacred ceremony originating from Ecuador, and practiced similarly in many other healing traditions around the world—in general, our North American society doesn't value the postpartum period or grief as sacred journeys, and there aren't many resources or rituals for the community. It's called *closing the bones*. She says that in this ceremony I will be honored deeply. Teresa is a death mid-wife, bereavement and loss doula, ritual healing practitioner, and celebrant, and she led the prenatal yoga classes I attended with both Reid and Everett.

With her guidance, she explains, I'll participate in the reclamation and restoration of my womb, heart, body, and soul—to respect my journey into motherhood. And through the rituals of this ceremony, the healing gestures of them, I will be guided and supported in honoring one of the greatest transitions in my life. In the literal act of closing the bones that have been altered to make space for this journey, and in a metaphorical sense to nurture the emotions that have embed-ded themselves within me as a result.

She asks me to lie down over the rebozos, long, straight pieces of cloth traditionally used in Mexico, used now by birth workers all over the world. Teresa shakes me gently, pulling the rebozos under me from side to side. First the one under my feet, then my hips, my chest, my head. She is drumming above me now, clearing energy with deep breaths and chant-ing a song in Sanskrit, one I recognize from her yoga classes. Music plays around us, growing louder and louder.

I see myself in flashes. Pregnant with Reid, then leaving him behind. Pregnant with Everett, then surrounded by fam-ily as he slept on my chest. Then, I see him lying lifeless in Aaron's arms in the hospital. I am crying and I don't know why. My whole body shakes from the weight of the sobs.

Out of nowhere, an image of my grandpa Patrick fills my mind. He leans over, kisses my forehead, and whispers, "You're alright now, kid." And I steady.

Teresa lures me into meditation with her voice. I am in nature. I see a four-legged friend, a speckled deer, hiding in the bushes. I realize I'm on the small island where our family owns property—no cars, remote and lush. Then I am walking along a path toward the base of a mountain edge, near the ocean. I see a door in the side of the mountain and I open it to enter. I follow a spiral staircase down and see crystals covering the walls. I notice their color, a rose hue. It takes me into a deep cave. And as I travel down to the very last step, listening to the sound of running water, I eventually come to a pond. I gaze into the reflection. Someone is there, but I can't see who. Through the ripples pulsing across the surface it almost looks like Everett.

I cup my hands together, dip them into the pond, and drink the fresh mountain water. Then I stand, turn, and see the figure. The face is covered now by a blood-red cloak. The hooded figure takes out a box and gives it to me. Inside there is a pendant. White, decorated with deep lines, like an open palm. I am meant to take it, so I fasten it to a chain and secure it around my neck.

The figure removes the hood. I still can't see his face, but it's Reid. I know.

Then Teresa is repeating, "You are here. You are here. You are here." And he is gone.

Slowly, I work my way out from the rebozos, which are bound up the length of my body, emerging from the cocoon woven around me. I move my legs and rotate my shoulders beneath the tension from the fabric. Finally, I am free. And though I understand that this act is meant to be a physical representation of the transformations I've experienced, I don't think I've gone from one state to another. It is more intricate than that.

I rest in child's pose for a while. Teresa burns palo santo wood, and a citrusy, sweet scent fills the air. As I release, sink further into the floor, white circles of light appear on the backs of my eyelids. I think I've made them up, until Teresa tells me she senses circles of support around me. Many generations coming together through my suffering. Starting at the center and expanding out, farther than she can see. And I remember—the kiss on my forehead, and the fact that it is two years to the day since my grandpa Patrick died.

It is curious. I am curious.

After Teresa closes the ceremony with me, we talk about my love for numbers. I admit that I scrolled through her Instagram, all the way to the beginning, and learned that her birthday is April 4 too. She places a palm over her heart. "You'll know, then. About forty-four?"

I raise my eyebrows. "No?"

"It is believed that the number forty-four means that angels are with us. Being born on the fourth day of the fourth month, this has always been significant to me," she explains.

I've always had a thing for numbers. I would find patterns and connections and meaning in them all around me. Often, while driving from one after-school activity to the next, my mom would play a game with me to pass the time. She would point out numbers—a license plate, a road sign, a random radio station—and ask if I could connect them to something significant. I always could, adding or subtracting or dividing to bend the numbers to my will. She was always surprised. I was always inspired. The poetry behind the numbers drew me in. It felt like magic.

Reid was born on April 4, 2015, at 2:24 AM: 4/4/15, 2:24. The first two numbers the same, the third different. Everett was born on December 16, 2016, at 6:44 PM: 12/16/16, 6:44. The first number different, the next two the same. Reid weighed 7 pounds, 11 ounces. Everett weighed 6 pounds, 12 ounces. The first number one less, the second number one more. Always the same pattern, the same blueprint, just reversed—mirror images. Like brothers.

Now, I consider the significance of the number forty-four. Reid's birthday, the fourth day of the fourth month: 44. His birth hour, 2:24 AM. Add the 2s, get 44 again. I do the math; Everett's birthday adds up to it too: 12+16+16 = 44. And he was born at 6:44 PM. What does it all mean, if anything at all?

Sometimes there is no explaining anything. No understanding, either. Maybe we aren't supposed to understand but instead trust our feelings. Maybe asking what it all means isn't the right question. Maybe all I need to ask is if it means something to me. Can that be enough?

Slowly, slowly, slowly, these bones that have shifted and broken wide open over the years are closing, though they will not stay this way forever. They are shifting to their new place of belonging, changed. I am learning how to have a relationship with one child that met death early on, and one that escaped it. Learning to love my life as it is, through the trauma and the hardships. I'm learning to love this world as it is, too. Because in this world, in these relationships and transitions and traumas, there is a softness like no other.

Not everyone needs to experience a ceremony with a celebrant or ritual-healing guide as I did, though they can. A guide offers a deep level of support. But I do think that in this lifetime that's full of transitions, we must find ways to process them, honor them, celebrate them. Feel everything that comes with them. Mark them with ceremony and ritual. We must invite others to experience them with us, in merriment and in grief. For the intimacies of death are too much to bear alone, and life is not meant to be lived alone anyway.

My transition into motherhood has transformed me. The metaphorical and literal deaths that have come with conceiving, growing, birthing, and raising my children have transformed me. And this transformation does not reduce my loss. Reid died, and beautiful things have happened through him. Not through his death, but through who he is.

20

A T THE TIME I am writing this, we are nearly three years
out from Reid's death. A sturdy, noisy, and wildly
observant little boy sits propped on my hip, joining
me in almost all that I do. We are moving forward with life
through the grief and anxiety of our past.

The ache of Grief is different now. No longer an ache
within an ache within an ache. It's no longer abstract but a
fully formed beast with pitchfork teeth and slimy skin and
a belly full of my dreams. And I still love him. Sometimes I
think I have him, this beast, and I draw him close and whisper,
"Hush now, don't fight." I think we are friends, that he might
love me too, that we are navigating a relationship that has
reached an understanding over the years. But then, suddenly,
Grief slips out from under my fingers and bites me hard on
the back of a thigh or a veiny arm or an exposed bit of neck.

I think I have a grasp on what I'm missing as Everett grows,
and I surrender to that longing daily. Then, something new.

Always something new. There are so many moments that I long to experience with Reid that I am experiencing with Everett now. It's the little ones that catch me by surprise, like the first discovery of lint on black tights. He picks it up with a precise pinch and extends the treasure out to me in absolute wonder, and I ache.

Just the other day, I balanced four tiny blocks with the letters of Reid's name above our full-length mirror. Everett looked up at them and laughed. He laughed! He reached his chubby fingers toward them and giggled. He quickly turned his head to me and smiled, then turned back to the blocks to reach for them again.

Of course, it could just be that he is a small child reacting to some new discovery, something he finds interesting. I don't live in that world anymore, though. Why would I want to? I live in a world where I am able to surrender to the reality that neither I nor any other living person knows what happens to a soul after death. Perhaps strangers see the light of traveling spirits and butterflies act in mysterious ways and little siblings' lives are saved due to intuition. Perhaps these things are possible because of the God that I know so very little about, but feel so intimately during the most unexpected times in my life.

But Reid is fading into my memory, and the visions of him are harder to bring forth with time. The edges of his face are blurry. I have the photos, but they're not the same. Although, often I come back to a single second, always the same one. One in which I forced myself to etch him into my mind. My arms still remember what the weight of him felt like, and sometimes they tingle in that specific way after a great weight has been removed. It's almost enough to bring me back. His skin, that mixture of pink and red and black. His swaddle, stained and wrinkled. His hat, slipping off the top of his head. Just as quickly the vision vanishes—that slippery beast—and I am left weeping for all the memories I didn't get with him instead of cherishing all the ones I did. It is easy to know to be grateful, but it's not always easy to know *how*.

If you look up the term "rainbow baby," you'll find that this is what a baby born following a miscarriage, stillbirth, or neo-natal death is called. Because after a storm ends a rainbow can appear, bringing promises of hope and calm and joy with it.

I appreciate the term, because it gives me an opportunity to tell my story in a softer way. If someone asks, "Is he your only child?" I can reply, "He is my rainbow baby." The mean-ing behind the term is an attractive one, because don't we all want to believe that even when awful things happen, happy endings are within reach? That rainbows exist? They do; I have seen them, lived inside of them.

That usual definition also makes me feel uncomfortable. Because it feeds into what we so wrongly perceive about grief: that there is an end to it. If the grief from Reid's loss is a storm and if that storm ended to make way for this rainbow, doesn't that imply that the pain of losing him ended too? Wouldn't that then mean that the love that made that grief possible was gone? We will *always* love our firstborn son. So we will always miss and grieve him. Nothing about Reid was like a storm, even though losing him was the hardest thing I've ever had to endure. But more than that, I count everything to do with him as a blessing. All while it hurts. All at the same time.

We could think about it in a different way. There doesn't need to be a storm, or its end, for there to be a rainbow, does there? Just rain and sun existing together. Sorrow and joy holding hands through the beauty of life and the pain of loss. For when we talk about a rainbow baby, we are integrating the one who came before them into our present. This is life and pregnancy and parenthood after loss.

● ☾ ●

I ACKNOWLEDGE FEAR every time I put Everett to sleep. When I get in the car with him. When we drive somewhere new. I imagine all of the different ways death may come, and try to stave it off. I watch his chest and I install a mirror and I buy a monitor. I google local hospitals and emergency rooms. I also know that one day, I will let these habits go, and he will live.

We are all, at any time, just one choice or encounter or action away from death. Aaron reminds me that while this is true, the opposite is as well: that we are all one choice or encounter or action away from life. The difference lies in how we choose to look at it. It is possible to live fully while we walk toward the deaths of our futures. And when death comes, for us or someone we love, we are able to live fully still. We honor the lives we have come to know, and we learn to carry them forward.

In her memoir *Let's Take the Long Way Home*, Gail Caldwell says: "dying doesn't end the story; it transforms it." I know she is right because death never ended the love I have for Reid, but it has changed how I express it. The tears of pain and words of remembering and marveling at signs are what that love looks like now. This is my grief.

On some level I have always known that grief and love were cut from the same cloth. There have been many moments of grace over the years, though they never quite had me moving forward—off a little to the side instead, or backward a touch. I have grown stronger and my grief has changed, but I'm only just beginning to feel like someone I can recognize as a whole human being, not shattered fragments of a wholly broken one.

Our fears are necessary for survival, but they can also be debilitating and paralyzing. They can own you. They have owned me. I have the opportunity to leave that fear-driven space now. Time and circumstance and work have all allowed for this. And only now does my healing feel real. Food isn't just fuel now—there's pleasure in it. Same with art or even conversations about a show on TV.

Aaron and I are able to laugh freely together again, and I see that the lines from frequent smiles are carving their way back into his face. Sex is intimate and passionate again too—it feels like love again—and if I'm being honest I'll admit it took years to get back to this place.

I know I'm healing because my perspective has changed. Where my focus was once on grieving for all I was missing of Reid, now I grieve for what Reid himself is missing. I am sad he isn't experiencing all that I wanted him to. Family dinners and vacations and birthday gifts. Now I mourn that he'll never get to do these things. My grief is no longer as selfish as it once was. There is room in my heart for more than just my own aches and pains.

● ☾ ●

I DRIVE BY a cemetery. I see the flowers left on top of the graves, evidence of relationships continuing, and I think about Reid and his ashes that sit on our desktop at home. But he's not there, not really. His life and legacy aren't tied to his body. Sometimes I reach out for something solid to pin my grief to, but I can never quite find it. Because he was never entirely here in the traditional way we understand people to be. Never entirely gone then, either.

I do ache for a physical place to go to when I want to be close to him, though. That's exactly what this book is; this is one of the forces driving me to complete it. It is my ceremony, my ritual. In it—in writing and sharing it—I am recognizing my motherhood journey as the sacred experience it's been. I am acknowledging that this story is significant, and that it is mine, and that others, millions of others, have similar ones to tell. It is in these stories where we find the love that remains.

I can return to these pages when I want to feel him near. Reid can rest in this book. He is in the words that tell of his ever-present soul, in all that he has and continues to inspire in me and in others. He is what I share of him and more.

There may not be a reason for everything that has happened in my life so far, but if there is, there will never be one that is good enough to warrant the death of my first child. And even if explanations exist, I cannot discover them during this lifetime, and it is nearly time to stop my crusade to seek them. But I can't ignore the connections and all that I've seen. There is too much for it all to simply be random—for everything to be a result of chaos and chance collisions. These inexplicable moments and revelations say to me: though terrible things happen, we are not left alone in them.

I don't believe that God caused Reid's death. I believe He is as heartbroken as I am. I believe that He leads me to find purpose in my suffering, but not to minimize it or elevate it to a "good" thing. Though I believe that good things can come out of loss—I have witnessed this firsthand. I believe He is helping me carry this suffering and providing me with the tools to see that life is hard—devastating even—and life is beautiful too. And so I no longer pray for changed outcomes, but for the grace and strength and comfort to let these outcomes change me.

I can smell the fall coming now, and it reminds me of my innocence. Despite all that's happened, I can still feel those tender youthful days and instead of pushing them away I embrace them, for they are part of me just as the tough memories are. And the scars of my past still open back up and weep sometimes, allowing the restorative cycle to continue.

This healing smells of asphalt, warming under that late-summer sun. It smells of sweat collecting above an upper lip. It seemed like sweater weather in the overcast morning, but then the clouds cleared to reveal a warmer day. And it smells of the early fallen leaves that crunch underfoot.

I wish Reid had lived. When I think back to it, I still will his heart to start beating. I stare at the screen in my mind where his heart is displayed at the center, unmoving, and I try to make it quiver, if only for a moment. But I cannot make it move. I can't change the way things really went. Even with all of the good that has filled my life since, I keep trying.

And I know that if Reid had lived, Everett wouldn't be here, and I can't imagine life without him either. I can't wrap my head around how all of this is true, how I can feel all of these things at once. And as my skin is kissed by the breeze, and Everett reaches a hand up toward me from the stroller as we walk, I melt, and I know, somehow, that everything is okay. Though the grief, *oh the grief,* it persists—growing and softening with everything this life after loss presents. Because this healing journey is always evolving, and it has no end.

I continue to push Everett through the autumn air, along the gravel path before us. He makes loud, drawn-out "Ahh!" noises, enjoying the way they vibrate as his stroller bounces over small rocks. Then, as the leaves whisper in the wind, he whispers back. Silent secrets exchanged between worlds. I wonder what he hears, and I smile knowing that one day I might ask him.

In the fading sunlight I catch a glimmer of red in his hair. But if I get too close, the illusion vanishes. There one minute and gone the next. Fading into that stretch of talking trees before us.

And if the red is there, how do I reconcile that with what has happened? With what is happening now? I don't. That his big brother's name should mean "red-haired" and that his hair has bits of the hue is one of those great unknowns in my life. Physical evidence of my internal, eternal longing. Still, even still, I'd like to understand. Just a little.

Notes

1. Reli Hershkovitz et al., "Risk Factors Associated with True Knots of the Umbilical Cord," *European Journal of Obstetrics & Gynecology and Reproductive Biology* 98, no. 1 (September 2001): 36–39, doi.org/10.1016/s0301-2115(01)00312-8.

2. Donald Winnicott and John Bowlby, quoted in Irvin D. Yalom and Molyn Leszcz, *Theory and Practice of Group Psychotherapy*, 5th ed. (New York: Basic Books, 2005), 20.

3. Joanne Cacciatore, "The Unique Experiences of Women and Their Families after the Death of a Baby," *Social Work in Health Care* 49, no. 2 (February 2010): 134–48, doi.org/10.1080/00981380903158078.

4. Ibid., 143.

5. Joy E. Lawn et al., "Stillbirths: Rates, Risk Factors, and Acceleration towards 2030," *The Lancet* 387, no. 10018 (February 6, 2016): 587–603, doi.org/10.1016/s0140-6736(15)00837-5.

6. "New 'Ending Preventable Stillbirths' *Lancet* Series—Accelerating Momentum in the Global Call to Action," International Stillbirth Alliance, accessed February 2019, stillbirthalliance. org/research/lancets-2016-stillbirths-series.

7. Some reported per-country stillbirth rates: Canada, 3.8/1000 (using a definition of ≥500 g); UK, 5.4/1000 (using a definition of ≥24 weeks); Australia, 2.9/1000 (using a definition of ≥28 weeks); US, 5.96/1000 (using a definition of ≥20 weeks); Pakistan, 43.1/1000 (using a definition of ≥28 weeks). Figures from Lawn, "Stillbirths: Rates," 587–603, and H. Blencowe et al., "National, Regional, and Worldwide Estimates of Stillbirth Rates in 2015, with Trends from 2000: A Systematic Analysis," *The Lancet* 4, no. 2 (February 1, 2016): e98–e108, doi: 10.1016/s2214-109x(15)00275-2. For US statistic: Marian F. MacDorman and Elizabeth C.W. Gregory, "Fetal and Perinatal Mortality: United States, 2013." *National Vital Statistics Reports* 64, no. 8 (July 23, 2015): 1.

8. Lawn, "Stillbirths: Rates," 587–603.

9. Dr. Vicki Flenady et al., "Stillbirths: Recall to Action in High-Income Countries," *The Lancet* 387, no. 10019 (February 13, 2016): 691–702, doi.org/10.1016/s0140-6736(15)01020-x.

10. Lawn, "Stillbirths: Rates," 587–603. The study identified twelve
    potentially modifiable risk factors for stillbirth, including
    demographics, such as maternal age ≥35; infections, such as
    syphilis, HIV, and malaria; noncommunicable disorders, such
    as overweight and obesity, maternal pre-existing diabetes,
    maternal pre-existing hypertension, pre-eclampsia, eclampsia,
    tobacco use; and fetal disorders, such as postterm pregnancy
    (≥42 weeks) and rhesus disease.

11. J. Muglu et al., "Risks of Stillbirth and Neonatal Death with
    Advancing Gestation at Term," *PLOS Medicine* 16, no. 7 (July
    2, 2019): e1002838, doi.org/10.1371/journal.pmed.1002838.

12. A. Sheppard et al., "Birth Outcomes among First Nations,
    Inuit and Métis Populations," *Health Reports*, Statistics
    Canada, November 15, 2017, www150.statcan.gc.ca/n1/
    pub/82-003-x/2017011/article/54886-eng.htm.

13. D. Nuzum, S. Meaney, and K. O'Donoghue, "The Pub-
    lic Awareness of Stillbirth: An Irish Population Study,"
    BJOG 125, no. 2 (January 2018): 246–52, ncbi.nlm.nih.gov/
    pubmed/28929637.

14. Janet Scott and Laura J. Price, "Women's Awareness of
    Stillbirth and Reaction to Messaging around Stillbirth
    Risk," abstract, *BMC Pregnancy and Childbirth* 17 (2017):
    1–47, bmcpregnancychildbirth.biomedcentral.com/
    articles/10.1186/s12884-017-1457-7.

15. Jane Warland, Georgie Beaufoy, and Jill Dorrian, "Giving Sleep Position Advice in Pregnancy: Will We Make Women Anxious?" abstract, *BMC Pregnancy and Childbirth* 17 (2017); 1–47.

16. Fran Boyle et al., "Care Practices after Stillbirth: An International Perspective," abstract, *BMC Pregnancy and Childbirth* 17 (2017): 1–47.

17. Francine deMontigny, Chantal Verdon, and Christine Gervais, "Assisting Health Professionals in Supporting Fathers after Stillbirth," abstract, *BMC Pregnancy and Childbirth* 17 (2017): 1–47.

18. Louise Stephens et al., "Improving Quality of Care in Pregnancies after Stillbirth—An Improvement Science Project in Two UK Maternity Hospitals," abstract, *BMC Pregnancy and Childbirth* 17 (2017): 1–47.

19. "What Is Stillbirth?" Centers for Disease Control and Prevention, last reviewed August 29, 2019, cdc.gov/ncbddd/stillbirth/facts.html.

20. Ying-Fen Tseng et al., "The Meaning of Rituals after a Stillbirth: A Qualitative Study of Mothers with a Stillborn Baby," *Journal of Clinical Nursing* 27, no. 5–6 (March 2018): 1134–42, doi.org/10.1111/jocn.14142.

21. M.M. Sisay et al., "A Qualitative Study of Attitudes and Values Surrounding Stillbirth and Neonatal Mortality among Grandmothers, Mothers, and Unmarried Girls in Rural Amhara and Oromiya Regions, Ethiopia: Unheard Souls in the Backyard,"

Journal of Midwifery & Women's Health 59, no. s1 (January/February 2014): s110–s117, doi: 10.1111/jmwh.12156.

22. Yaira Hamama-Raz, Hadas Hartman, and Eli Buchbinder, "Coping with Stillbirth among Ultraorthodox Jewish Women," *Qualitative Health Research* 24, no. 7 (June 3, 2014): 923–32, doi.org/10.1177/1049732314539568.

23. Maureen L. Walsh, "Emerging Trends in Pregnancy-Loss Memorialization in American Catholicism," *Horizons* 44, no. 2 (December 2017): 369–98, doi.org/10.1017/hor.2017.63.

Acknowledgments

THE LIST OF those I owe gratitude to for both the physical creation of this book and the living of its tales is a long one, and yet I am sure that I will miss someone. So to all the written and unwritten contributors, guides, and inspirations in my life: thank you.

To Rob Sanders, founder of Greystone Books, thank you for your faith in my ability to tell this story. For giving me, a first-time author, an opportunity to publish this book and share my story with others.

To Paula Ayer, my editor turned friend, my sounding board. You have navigated the difficult task of analyzing a life story with such awareness and compassion. Your ability to offer critique and advice on the most intimate portrayals of my life has been a gift, and has helped me to understand more about my experiences in the process.

To Nancy Flight, my very first editor, I am grateful for your early insight that shaped the vision for this book. To Antonia Banyard, thank you for your counsel during the copyediting. To everyone else at Greystone Books, I am deeply appreciative of all that you've done to help bring this memoir to life.

To my Instagram and blog communities. *You* have made this book possible. If you hadn't instilled bravery in me as you so courageously shared your own losses, if I didn't have a compassionate place to share my journey, this story may never have been told. Thank you for receiving me during my darkest days and carrying me through to my joy.

To everyone who contributed their knowledge and expertise to strengthen the areas beyond my scope, thank you. To Teresa of La Lupa Via, I extend immeasurable gratitude to you and your selflessness, for holding space for my grief, for encouraging my curiosity, for providing insight into how to be more inclusive with words as well as heart, and for speaking the truth you so fiercely believe in with such grace. It is an honor to know you. To Andrew, for providing insight into the world of psychotherapy. To Dr. F., for your compassionate heart and willingness to educate me on the world of stillbirth studies and bereavement care.

To Amy, thank you for saying Reid's name, without fail, every single time we meet. Thank you for wrestling with me through all of the hard questions. To Brittany, thank you for journeying with me into motherhood, and thank you for answering the phone. To Amelia, for creating space for healing with Landon's Legacy Retreat. I am grateful for your friendship and the insight you have given me in this new normal we find ourselves navigating. To the women I met at Landon's Legacy Retreat, for being a constant source of support.

To the parents of the club of the bereaved that I have come to know and love over the years, thank you for truly seeing me and for teaching me how to see in return. To the children I believe are keeping Reid company: Madison (Amrit), Evan (Kathy), Florence (Michaela), Lochlan (Katie), Joseph (Jenna), Landon (Amelia), Benedict (Jennifer), Aby (Maria Elena), Paisley (Jessica), Bo (Karin), Aubrey (Savanna), Liam (Jackie), Makinsie (Jude), Henry (Laura), Emma (Tiffany), Aedan (Krista), Zelda (Amanda), Greyson (Jenna), Halyn (Brooke), Jack (Katharine), Madisyn (Darcy), Millie (Lissa), RJ (Christine), Isabella (Alexandra), Luisa (Julia), Enya (Kaiti), Sophie (Wardy), Saul (Kimberly), and those not named here who are remembered always. Each and every one of you have a place in my heart.

To the medical staff of BC Women's Hospital and BC Children's Hospital: thank you for your outstanding care during my pregnancies and the births of both my children, for the bereavement care after Reid's death, for saving Everett's life and nurturing him to strength after. To Sam, Everett's nurse, for advocating so fiercely for us, and for providing insight into the medical details of that experience as I wrote about them. To our doula, Jill, for supporting us through the physical, physiological, and emotional aspects of both birth and death. To our midwife, Susie, thank you for being the first person to welcome me into this terrible and somehow wonderful club of the bereaved. For sharing about your son Isaac. For showing me, above all, that there *is* life after loss. To Dr. B., you fostered the care necessary to ensure that Everett would arrive safely in our arms. You went above and beyond with your love, your humor, your straight talking, your knowledge of how to care for me. I could not have endured all that came with pregnancy after loss if it weren't for you. To the midwives, family physicians, ultrasound technicians, nurses, receptionists, social workers, chaplain, obstetricians: I cannot name you all, but I hope you know the invaluable role you have played in our journey, and how far-reaching our love for you is.

To my VandenBrink family, immediate and extended: Annette, Hank, Hanah, Carson, Derek, Angela, Levi, Katie, I thank you for your open-mindedness, for your grace that allowed me to write about how our lives are connected. Thank you for all the ways you keep Reid alive with your words and actions.

To those who met Reid's physical body: Aaron, Mom, Dad, Alana, Milan, Rebecca, Trenton, Grandma, Annette, Hank, Hanah, Carson, Micaela. We are a small group that shared in a sacred experience and I am grateful for all of you.

To family and friends for giving your time to hang out with Everett so that I could enter the headspace necessary to write this book. Rebecca, Alana, Dad, Aaron, Hanah, Hank, thank you. And thank you to my mother-in-law, Annette, and my mother, Amanda, especially—I am indebted to you both and so eternally grateful for the generous gifts of your time. This book would not have been completed without this tremendous act of support from each and every one of you, named and not named.

To Hanah and Micaela, for your friendship, patience, support, and continued presence in my life. And for your shared love of memes and good, strong coffee. I cherish our sisterhood, and I don't know what I would do or where I would be without either of you.

To my sisters, Alana and Rebecca, for your unconditional love that has grown over the years into a bond like no other, connecting us as both family and friends. Thank you for supporting me every step of the way. I love you, and I love the way you love your nephews.

To my grandmother, Alison, without whom I am entirely sure I would not have agreed to embark on the journey of writing this book. You instilled a love of reading in me from a very young age—standing in lines for new releases, taking me to readings by my favorite authors, and helping me grow my personal library. Thank you for nurturing me as a writer, for that day you and Grandpa said, "You'll publish a book one day, my dear."

To my mother and father, for reading this manuscript in its earliest form, braving the incredible pain that reliving these memories caused, and turning it into the inspiration I needed. Thank you for opening your home to our family, and for allowing Everett to experience the best of all of us as a result.

To Mom, thank you for mothering me during this time when I needed to be mothered the most. I have never longed for your care, or required it at such depths, as I have since I became a mother. Thank you for the practical things: the long walks in search of new homes, the food, the laundry. Thank you for the essential ones: the conversations, the time spent together, the sleepovers. For showing me how to add color to my parenting.

To Dad, thank you for teaching me in actions more than words what it is to create meaning out of suffering. For the late nights we spent talking about God and reasons and randomness. For the counsel you provided on the big questions I wrestled with in writing this memoir, and for showing me that the whys are not as important as I think.

To Aaron, my best friend, my lover, my partner in this life. This is not quite what we imagined when we first met all those years ago, but there's no one else I'd rather be navigating it with. Thank you for all of the times you carried me as well as yourself, for your support in real time as we lived these moments and after as I wrote and edited them for the eyes of readers. P.S. I love you.

To Atticus, the son who entered our story in the final months of editing this manuscript. My love, though you are not written on these pages, this is your story too, and you influenced many of the changes I made at the end. Thank you for keeping me company with your kicks and rolls as I revised it to completion.

To Everett, you are my reason, my motivation for publishing this book. I dream of your future world that holds space for real, raw, honest conversations about life and the heartaches that are a part of it. My love and hopes for you are woven into this work. Thank you for understanding that the time I needed to take to write this was not time away from you, but instead time with your big brother. You are a bright light in the lives of many. You are my greatest teacher.

To Reid, this is for you. I feel you all around; in the fullness of the moon or on significant dates. Your presence in our family lives on. Still, I miss you every single day. And I love you. Until we meet again, I will spend my life trying to honor you and further your legacy. Thank you for making me a mother.

Recommended Reading

I N ADDITION TO the scientific studies I examined while writing this book, I turned to memoirs, books on the psychology of grief, poetry, and fiction. Many of the works listed on the following pages served as important guides in my personal journey with grief, and my wish in sharing this list is that it might also help those who are currently mourning, those supporting the bereaved, and those who will experience loss in their futures.

MEMOIRS

Ask Me His Name: Learning to Live and Laugh Again after the Loss of My Baby by Elle Wright

Blue Nights by Joan Didion

The Bright Hour: A Memoir of Living and Dying by Nina Riggs

Brother, I'm Dying by Edwidge Danticat

Comfort: A Journey through Grief by Ann Hood

Dead Babies and Seaside Towns by Alice Jolly

Disaster Falls: A Family Story by Stéphane Gerson

Everything Happens for a Reason: And Other Lies I've Loved by Kate Bowler

An Exact Replica of a Figment of My Imagination by Elizabeth McCracken

A Grief Observed by C.S. Lewis

Hannah's Gift: Lessons from a Life Fully Lived by Maria Housden

It's Okay to Laugh (Crying Is Cool Too) by Nora McInerny Purmort

Landon's Legacy: The Power of a Brief Life by Amelia Kathryn Barnes

Let's Take the Long Way Home: A Memoir of Friendship by Gail Caldwell

The Long Goodbye: A Memoir by Meghan O'Rourke

Once More We Saw Stars: A Memoir by Jayson Greene

Poor Your Soul by Mira Ptacin

Rare Bird: A Memoir of Loss and Love by Anna Whiston-Donaldson

The Rules Do Not Apply: A Memoir by Ariel Levy

This Is Happy: A Memoir by Camilla Gibb

When Breath Becomes Air by Paul Kalanithi

The Year of Magical Thinking by Joan Didion

FICTION

Grief Is the Thing with Feathers by Max Porter

Swimmer in the Secret Sea by William Kotzwinkle

POETRY

The Art of Losing: Poems of Grief and Healing by Kevin Young

Poems of Mourning by Peter Washington

GRIEF EDUCATION

Bearing the Unbearable: Love, Loss, and the Heartbreaking Path of Grief by Joanne Cacciatore

Getting Grief Right: Finding Your Story of Love in the Sorrow of Loss by Patrick O'Malley

It's OK That You're Not OK: Meeting Grief and Loss in a Culture That Doesn't Understand by Megan Devine

On Grief and Grieving: Finding the Meaning of Grief through the Five Stages of Loss by Elisabeth Kübler-Ross

The Unspeakable Loss: How Do You Live after a Child Dies? by Nisha Zenoff

---

Visit www.emmahansen.ca for updated and additional resources, including current links to relevant websites and social media accounts, and guides for the grieving and their loved ones. Connect with Emma on her Instagram: @emmahansen